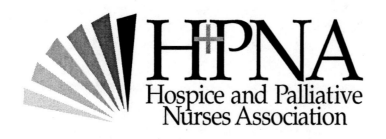

CORE CURRICULUM FOR THE GENERALIST HOSPICE AND PALLIATIVE NURSE

Coordinating Editors:

Barbara G. Volker, RN, MSN, CHPN
Consultant/Educator—Hospice/Palliative Care
Volker Consulting Service
Fresno, California

Ashby C. Watson, RN, MS, CS, OCN
Psychosocial Oncology Clinical Nurse Specialist
MCV Hospitals and Physicians of the Virginia
Commonwealth University Health System
Richmond, Virginia

KENDALL/HUNT PUBLISHING COMPANY
4050 Westmark Drive   Dubuque, Iowa 52002

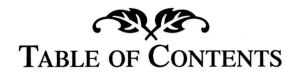

TABLE OF CONTENTS

CHAPTER IV: PATIENT CARE: PAIN MANAGEMENT

CHAPTER V: SYMPTOM MANAGEMENT

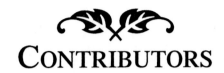

CONTRIBUTORS

Terry Altilio, ACSW
Social Work Coordinator
Department of Pain Medicine and Palliative
  Care
Beth Israel Medical Center
New York, NY

Patricia H. Berry, PhD, APRN-BC, CHPN
Assistant Professor
College of Nursing
University of Utah
Salt Lake City, UT

Cathleen A. Collins, RN, MSN, CHPN
Instructor of Clinical Nursing
Texas Tech University Health Sciences Center
School of Nursing
Lubbock, TX

Constance Dahlin, MSN, RNCS, CHPN, ANP
Palliative Care Nurse Practitioner
Palliative Care Service
Massachusetts General Hospital
Boston, MA

Judith B. Eighmy, RN, BSN, CHPN
Partner, Pacific Healthcare Consultants
Rolling Hills Estates, CA

Betty Rolling Ferrell, Ph.D., FAAN
Research Scientist
Department of Nursing Education and
  Research
City of Hope National Medical Center
Duarte, CA

Kathy Kalina, RN, BSN
Support System Specialist
Center for Learning
Texas Health Resources
Arlington, TX

Marianne LaPorte Matzo, Ph.D., RN, CS
Graduate College Core Faculty
The Union Institute
Cincinnati, OH

Patricia Murphy, RN, MA
Chief Executive Officer
Hospice of Martin & St. Lucie
Stuart, FL

Elayne J. Nahman, LCSW, ACSW
Partner, Pacific Healthcare Consultants
Rolling Hills Estates, CA

Judith A. Paice, Ph.D., RN, FAAN
Research Professor of Medicine
Palliative Care and Home Hospice Program
Northwestern Memorial Hospital
Northwestern University
Chicago, IL

Molly Poleto, BSN, RN, CHPN
Consultant
Delmar, NY

Ellen C. Rooney, RNC, BSN
Hospice Nursing and Education Consultant
Fredericksburg, VA

Joanne E. Sheldon, RN, M.Ed, CHPN, CIC
Education Coordinator of the Hospice Institute
Hospice of the Western Reserve
Euclid, OH

Lizabeth H. Sumner, RN, BSN
Director, Children's Program
San Diego Hospice
Vista, CA

Barbara G. Volker, RN, MSN, CHPN (Editor)
Consultant/Educator—Hospice and
    Palliative Care
Volker Consulting Service
Fresno, CA

Ashby C. Watson, RN, MS, CS, OCN (Editor)
Psychosocial Oncology Clinical Nurse
    Specialist
MCV Hospitals & Physicians of the Virginia
    Commonwealth University Health System
Richmond, VA

Margery A. Wilson, MSN, FNP, CHPN
Palliative Care Nurse Practitioner
Wellmont Health System
Bristol, TN

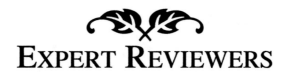

EXPERT REVIEWERS

Gail B. Aaron, RN, BSN, CHPN
Director, The Palliative Care Service
Providence Hospital
Washington, DC

Laurie J. Cooksey, Pharm.D.
MCV Hospitals & Physicians of the Virginia
    Commonwealth University Health System
Richmond, VA

Nessa Coyle, MSN, RN, FAAN
Director of the Supportive Care Program
Palliative Care Service
Memorial Sloan-Kettering Cancer Center
New York, NY

Patrick J. Coyne, RN, MSN, CS, CHPN
Clinical Nurse Specialist
MCV Hospitals & Physicians of the Virginia
    Commonwealth University Health System
Richmond, VA

Constance Dahlin, MSN, RN, ANP
Advanced Practice Palliative Care Nurse
Massachusettes General Hospital
Boston, MA

Betty Davies, RN, Ph.D., FAAN
Professor and Chair
Department of Family Health Care Nursing
School of Nursing
University of California—San Francisco
San Francisco, CA

Kathleen Egan, MA, BSN, CHPN
Vice President
Hospice Institute of the Florida Suncoast
Largo, FL

Julie Griffie RN, MSN, CS, AOCN
Palliative Care Advanced Practice Nurse
Medical College of Wisconsin
Milwaukee, WI

Judy Lentz, RN, MSN, OCN, NHA
Executive Director, HPNA
Pittsburgh, PA

Susan McMillen, PHD, ARNP, FAAN
USF College of Nursing
Tampa, FL

Elizabeth G. Miller, RD
MCV Hospitals & Physicians of the Virginia
    Commonwealth University Health System
Richmond, VA

Pat Murphy, PhD, APN, FAAN
Patient Care Services
UMDNJ University Hospital
Newark, NJ

Elizabeth Ford Pitorak MSN, RN, CHPN
Director, Hospice Institute
Hospice of the Western Reserve
Cleveland, OH

Molly Poleto, BSN, RN, CHPN
Consultant
Delmar, NY

Susan Riddell, MS, RN, NHA
Administrator
Mariner HealthCare
Palm City, FL

Mary Robinson, RN, MS, CRNH, CHT
Director of Nursing
Triangle Hospice
Durham, NC

Shirley A. Smith, RN, MSN, CRNH
Hospice Educator and Consultant
Dallas, PA

Jan Wendt, RN, MA, CRNH
Director of Edcuation/Research
HPNA
Pittsburgh, PA

Marie Whedon, MSN, RN, CHPN
Norris Cotton Cancer Center
Dartmouth-Hitchcock Medical Center
Lebanon, NH

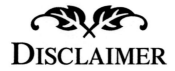

DISCLAIMER

The Hospice and Palliative Nurses Association,
its officers and directors and the authors and
reviewers of this core curriculum make no claims
that buying or studying it will guarantee a passing
score on the CHPN Certification examination.

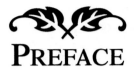

PREFACE

The development of this *Core Curriculum for the Generalist Hospice and Palliative Nurse* has been a long journey, one that began when nurses preparing to take the first hospice nurse certification examination in 1994 requested materials to review. These requests led to the development of the *Hospice Nurses Certification Exam Review: A Self-Study Guide* by Ken Zeri, Kathleen Egan and Virginia Shubert (1994). That first effort was followed in 1997 by a second edition, *The Hospice Nurse's Study Guide: A Preparation for the CRNH Candidate* by Patricia Berry, Ken Zeri and Kathleen Egan.

In 1999, *The Hospice Nurses Study Guide* was transformed into the *Hospice and Palliative Nursing Practice Review* with the work of eleven contributors edited by Barbara Volker. While the book was based on the certification test outline content, hospices and palliative care services began using it to establish a basic level of nursing knowledge in end of life care. This indicated the need for a more comprehensive, referenced and current didactic review of the core components of care in the hospice and palliative specialty.

The *Core Curriculum for the Generalist Hospice and Palliative Nurse* is intended not only for hospice and palliative nurses but also for nurses in other practice settings. The information and resources in this curriculum can be of benefit to any nurse whose clients have a life-limiting progressive illness. The curriculum includes an expanded end of life content with additional chapters on pediatric end of life care, on the challenges of providing end of life care for patients who are in more traditional settings, and on economic issues and trends in the field.

Many in hospice nursing have seen the parallels between hospice nursing and nursing in the labor and delivery setting. A contributing author, Kathy Kalina, wrote a book called *Midwife for Souls: Spiritual Care for the Dying* (1993) that is a pastoral guide for hospice workers and those who live with the terminally ill. In it, she comments on the symmetry between natural birth and natural death.

As we began work on this curriculum, we looked at the current written materials, at information we wanted to add and, as hospice and palliative nurses often do, considered the journey that begins for any family when one of its members is diagnosed with a life-limiting progressive illness. Our discussions focused particularly on that journey and we came to the conclusion that the curriculum should follow a similar progression. Thus we begin with the history and development of the hospice and palliative care movements and of the Interdisciplinary Team; move to patterns of disease progression and management of pain and other symptoms, discuss indicators of imminent death; and finish by looking at economic issues and trends for the future.

A project of this scope would be impossible without the help of people too numerous to mention. We gratefully acknowledge all of those authors who contributed to the study guides and the practice review that preceded this work. They laid the strong foundation upon which we built the curriculum. Thanks are also due to the writers and reviewers of this book from the disciplines of hospice, palliative care, pharmacy, and dietary counseling. Their names and credentials are listed. We owe a special debt of gratitude to Connie Dahlin, Chair of the HPNA Education/Research Committee and Judy Lentz, Executive Director of HPNA. Their patience and support throughout this process has been remarkable. Finally, we wish to acknowledge and thank our families. A work such as this takes much time and effort. We could not have completed it without their love and support.

Barbara G. Volker, RN, MSN, CRNH
Ashby Watson, RN, MS, CS, OCN
Editors

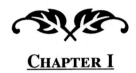

CHAPTER I

AN OVERVIEW OF HOSPICE AND PALLIATIVE CARE

Barbara G. Volker, RN, MSN, CHPN
Ashby C. Watson, RN, MS, CS, OCN

I. **History of Hospice and Palliative Care**

A. **Hospice**

1. Concept antedates 475 AD

2. The term "hospes," from which the term hospice is derived, means to be both host and guest; implies an interaction and mutual caring between patient, family, and hospice staff

3. Self-sustained communities evolved after 335 AD where ill, weary, homeless, and dying persons received care

4. During the early middle ages, words *hospice, hospital,* and *hostel* were used interchangeably

5. Also during the middle ages *hospitia*, or traveler's rests provided food, shelter, as well as care for those sick or dying

6. The care and support of the whole person (the soul, mind, spirit) evolved in these early hospices

7. Evolved to care for the sick and incurables in 1800's

8. The word hospice became synonymous with care of the terminally ill late in the 1800's with the founding of Our Lady's Hospice in Dublin by Sister May Aikenhead of the Irish Sisters of Charity, who was a colleague of Florence Nightingale

9. St. Joseph's Hospice established in 1900 in London; Dame Cicely Saunders began refining the ideas and protocols that form the cornerstone of modern hospice care in the 1950's and 60's

10. Cicely Saunders, MD opened St. Christopher's Hospice in 1960's in suburban London, marking the beginning of the modern hospice movement

11. Cicely Saunders, MD visited the US in 1963 and spoke to the medical and nursing students, and interested others at Yale University

12. Florence Wald, Dean of Yale School of Nursing, resigned to plan and found the Connecticut Hospice

13. The Palliative Care service at the Royal Victoria Hospital, Montreal, Canada, started by Balfour Mount, MD opened in 1975; first use of the term "palliative care" to refer to a program of care for terminally ill persons and their families; this became the first hospice in North America

14. The Connecticut Hospice incorporated in 1971, began seeing home care patients in 1974, 44 bed inpatient facility opened in 1979; the first hospice in the US

15. 1983 Tax Equity Fiscal Responsibility Act created the Medicare Hospice Benefit; defines hospice care in the US

B. Palliative Care

1. David Tasma, a Polish Jew who died of cancer in a London hospital in 1948—left Cicely Saunders a small legacy, saying, "I want to be a window in your home."

2. She acknowledges her interaction with him as the beginning of her work with thousands of dying patients, from which she established science of palliative medicine:

   a) Attends to the whole person

   b) Is limited to those who have progressive predictable disease

   c) Uses scientific rigor in developing treatment for pain and symptoms[1]

3. Contrasting views exist about the evolution of palliative care:

   a) Hospice and palliative care are often seen as synonymous, e.g., in England and Canada, hospice is also called palliative care[2]

   b) Hospice is thought to be a subset of palliative care[3]

   c) Palliative care found its roots in hospice[4]

   d) Hospice includes the elements of palliative care, but not all palliative care includes all the elements of hospice care[5]

II. Development of Modern Hospice and Palliative Care Movements

A. Hospice landmark events

1. Development of current concepts of palliative care are, in large part, through the work of Dame Cicely Saunders at St. Christopher's Hospice in London, including the use of scheduled oral opioids for pain management

2. Elisabeth Kubler-Ross's work in the 1960's demystified death and dying and opened the debate on care of the dying for health care professionals and the lay public; *On Death and Dying* was published in 1969

3. Increased knowledge and research regarding grief, loss, and bereavement

4. General dissatisfaction (among the public and some factions of the health care system) about how dying persons and their families are treated in the US health care system which generally emphasizes technological intervention and over treatment to prevent death

5. Development of the holistic nursing practice model

6. Issues related to cost of care versus quality of life

7. Physician assisted suicide movement and the 1995 results of the SUPPORT study, showing high incidence of uncontrolled pain (from 74% to 95%) in very ill and dying adults in spite of planned interventions from nurses to encourage physicians to attend to pain control[6]

8. The "natural death" consumer movement similar to the natural childbirth movement

9. Publication by the National Hospice Organization (NHO) of *A Pathway for Patients and Families Facing Terminal Illness* (1997)

10. Development by the National Hospice and Palliative Care Organization (NHPCO) of *Hospice Standards of Practice* (2001)

B. Palliative Care

1. Major factors have influenced the recent development of palliative care programs in the United States:

   a) Consumer demand

      (1) Aging of the population

      (2) Growing public interest in assisted suicide and euthanasia

      (3) Growing gap between what people with life-threatening illness desire and what they experience from health care systems and providers

      (4) Supreme Court's ruling on the right to die and its affirmation of right to care at the end of life

   b) Acknowledgment by medical community that care of dying is poor

      (1) SUPPORT Study results[6]

      (2) Institute of Medicine's report on End of Life Care (1997)

      (3) Development of WHO Standards for Cancer Pain Relief (1996)

      (4) WHO guidelines on Cancer Pain Relief and Palliative Care (1990)

      (5) AHCPR Cancer Pain Guidelines (now Agency for Healthcare Research and Quality [AHRQ])

      (6) Grassroots development of State Cancer Pain Initiatives (now American Alliance of Cancer Pain Initiatives)

      (7) Efforts of Project on Death in America, LAST ACTS Initiative, and Center to Improve the Care of the Dying[7]

      (8) Americans for Better Care of the Dying (ABCD)

      (9) Center for Palliative Care (CAPC)

III. Hospice Philosophy

A. Definitions of hospice

1. Medicare describes hospice as: an approach to caring for terminally ill individuals that stresses palliative care (relief of pain and uncomfortable symptoms), as opposed to curative care. In addition to meeting the patient's medical needs, hospice care addresses the physical, psychosocial, and spiritual needs of the patient, as well as the psychosocial needs of the patient's family/caregiver. The emphasis of the hospice program is on keeping the hospice patient at home with family and friends as long as possible

2. The National Hospice and Palliative Care Organization (NHPCO) describes hospice as a specialized form of multidisciplinary health care which is designed to provide palliative care, alleviate the physical, emotional, social and spiritual discomforts of an individual who is experiencing the last phase of life due to the existence of a life-limiting, progressive disease, to provide supportive care to the primary care giver and the family of the hospice patient

3. Hospice and Palliative Nurses Association (HPNA) defines hospice nursing as the provision of palliative nursing care for the terminally ill and their families with the emphasis on their physical, psychosocial, emotional, and spiritual needs. This care is accomplished in collaboration with an interdisciplinary team through a service that is available 24 hours a day, 7 days a week. The service comprises pain and symptom management, bereavement and volunteer components. Hospice nursing, then, is holistic practice conducted within an affiliative matrix. The hospice nurse, in developing and maintaining collaborative relationships with other members of the interdisciplinary team, must be flexible in dealing with the inevitable role blending that takes place. In functioning as a case manager, coordinating the implementation of the interdisciplinary team developed plan of care, the hospice nurse also shares an advocacy role for patients and their families with other members of the team

B. Key concepts in hospice philosophy

1. The patient and family (as defined by the patient) are considered the single unit of care

2. Hospice uses a core interdisciplinary team to address the physical, social, emotional, and spiritual needs of the patient and family

3. Hospice provides for the medical treatment of pain and other distressing symptoms associated with the life-limiting, progressive illness, but does not provide interventions to cure the disease or prolong life

4. The interdisciplinary team develops the overall plan of care, in accordance with the wishes of the patient and family, in order to provide coordinated care that emphasizes supportive services such as home care, pain management and limited inpatient services

5. Hospice care actively engages the community by utilizing volunteer support in delivering hospice services

6. The patient's home, or place of primary residence no matter where that may be (skilled nursing or residential care facilities, prisons, shelters, daycare centers for the elderly, etc.), is the primary site of hospice care

7. The philosophy of hospice emphasizes comfort, dignity and quality of life, with the focus on spiritual and existential issues throughout dying, death and bereavement

8. Patients and families are empowered to achieve as much control over their lives as possible

C. Desired goals for end of life care [8]

1. Self-determined life closure: terminally ill patients who are mentally competent should have freedom to decide how the rest of their life is spent within the options allowed by law

2. Safe and comfortable dying: patients are able to die free of distressing symptoms

3. Effective grieving: surviving family members/significant others are supported through the normal grieving process

D. Issues for Hospice

1. Six months life expectancy or less may be seen as death sentence by some physicians who thus may be reluctant to refer to hospice

2. Insurers may not pay for high-tech care and may limit access to specialists

3. Physicians may be reluctant to discuss Do Not Resuscitate (DNR) orders; patient and family may not be ready to accept them although DNR orders are not required for hospice admission

4. Referrals often occur when death is imminent, thus rushing hospice to quickly bond with family and initiate symptom management in crisis mode

5. Significant barriers to the management of pain continue to exist

IV. Philosophy of Palliative Care

A. Definitions of Palliative Care

1. The National Hospice Organization (NHO, 1988) defined palliative care as treatment that enhances comfort and improves quality of life. *No specific therapy is excluded from consideration.* The test of palliative treatment lies in the agreement by the patient, the physician, the family or primary caregiver, and the hospice team that the expected outcome is relief from distressing symptoms, easing of pain, and enhancement of quality of life

2. The active total care of patients whose disease is not responsive to curative treatment when control of pain, of other symptoms and of psychological, social, and spiritual problems is paramount. The goal of palliative care is the best possible quality of life for patients and their families[9]

3. Philosophy of care that provides a combination of active and compassionate therapies intended to support and comfort individuals and families who are living with life threatening illness, being sensitive and respectful of their religious, cultural, and personal beliefs, values and traditions[10]

4. Palliative care is defined as "...the prevention and relief of suffering through the management of symptoms from the early through the final stages of an illness" and "...attends closely to the emotional, spiritual, and practical needs/goals of the patient/family with life-threatening disease across the illness, dying trajectory"[11]

B. **Key concepts of Palliative Care philosophy[12]**

1. Affirms life and regards dying as a normal process that is neither hastened nor postponed

2. Provides relief from pain and other distressing symptoms

3. Integrates the psychological and spiritual aspects of patient care

4. Offers a support system to help the family cope during the patient's illness and their own bereavement

C. **Precepts of Palliative Care according to the Last Acts Initiative, 1998**

1. Respect for patient goals, preferences, and choices

2. Comprehensive care

    a) Addresses holistic needs

    b) Alleviates isolation

    c) Commits to ongoing communication and non-abandonment

3. Utilizes strengths of interdisciplinary resources

4. Acknowledges/addresses caregiver concerns and desire for supportive services

5. Develops institutional infrastructures that support best practices and best models of palliative care

6. Excellent interdisciplinary team coordination among all care giving environments

7. Focus of care based on patient and family values, addresses holistic growth and healing

8. Care is flexible, e.g., curative, palliative, or preventive in focus

D. **Core Principles of Palliative Care**

1. Family is the unit of care

2. Meaning of disease, suffering, life and death are addressed within each unique family unit

3. Commitment to collaboration through team process

4. Ethical principles of care are incorporated into daily practice

E. **Issues for Palliative Care**

1. Patients, families and staff may have difficulty transitioning from curative to palliative care

2. Most programs are located in hospital-based, hierarchical medical institutions

3. Some programs may not provide continuity and communication with primary care physicians and community-based programs

4. Some programs may not provide supportive services, such as social work, spiritual, volunteer or bereavement follow-up

V. Hospice Care in the United States*

A. Programs

1. There are approximately 3,100 operational hospice programs in all 50 states, Puerto Rico and Guam

2. Most states (44 as of 1999) have hospice licensure laws that define specific requirements for operating as a hospice program

B. Patients

1. In 2000, nearly 2.4 million Americans died. In the same year an estimated 600,000 patients died while under the care of a hospice

2. Hospice programs were involved in providing care for approximately 25 percent of Americans who died from all causes in 2000

C. Reimbursement

1. Medicare: Many hospices are Medicare certified; in 1997 Medicare spent about $2 billion of its $200 billion budget on hospice services for 382,989 patients

2. Medicaid: Hospice is covered under Medicaid in 43 states and the District of Columbia

3. Private insurance: Most private insurance plans include a hospice benefit; 82% of managed care plans offer hospice services; coverage for hospice is available to more than 80% of employees in medium and large size businesses

D. Organizational structure and admission patterns

1. Ownership:

   a) 43% free-standing entities

   b) 33% division of hospital

   c) 22% division of home health agency

   d) 9% managed care providers

   e) 8% other

2. Financial designation:

   a) 73% nonprofit

   b) 20% for-profit

   c) 7% government organizations

---

* Data is from the National Hospice and Palliative Care Organization, Facts and Figures on Hospice Care in America, November 8, 2001.

E.   Accreditation

    1.   There is currently no mandatory nationwide certification or accreditation for hospices

    2.   In 2000, 91% of all hospices were Medicare certified and 62% of hospices were accredited

F.   Patient information

    1.   Diagnosis:

        a)   57% cancer

        b)   10% end-stage heart disease

        c)   6% dementia

        d)   6% lung disease

        e)   3% end-stage kidney disease

        f)   2% end-stage liver disease

    2.   Average length of enrollment in 2000 was 48 days; median length of stay was 25 days

    3.   78% of hospice patients died in their residence or under hospice care in a nursing home

    4.   In 2000, 82% of hospice patients were White or Caucasian; 8% Black or African American; 2% Hispanic or Latino; 2% identified as "other"; 6% not classified in any category

G.   Cost savings and revenue

    1.   For every dollar Medicare spends on hospice, $1.52 is saved

    2.   In the last year of life, hospice patients on the Medicare hospice benefit incurred approximately $2,737 less in costs than those not on the Medicare hospice benefit; savings totaled $3,192 in the last month of life

    3.   In 1995 hospices received revenue from the following sources: Medicare, 74%; private insurance, 12%; Medicaid 7%; and other, including donations, grants, private pay, 7%

VI.   Palliative Care in the United States*

A.   Programs

    1.   1st formal program was St. Luke's in New York City started in 1970's, relied on philanthropic support

        a)   Comprehensive interdisciplinary team saw patients in the ER and on nursing units

        b)   Closed in mid 1980's for lack of support

---

* Data is from "Pioneer Programs in Palliative Care: Nine Case Studies", Milbank Memorial Fund, New York: 2000.

2. A number of palliative care services have recently opened;
    similarities and differences include:

    a) Payor sources

    b) Funding sources

    c) Diagnoses

    d) Research and grant funding sources

    e) Organizational/administrative structure

    f) Programs offered

    g) Revenue/cost savings projected/reported

3. Nine pioneer palliative care programs have been developed.

    a) Balm of Gilead Center, Cooper Green Hospital, Birmingham, Alabama

    b) Palliative Care Programs, Beth Israel Deaconess Medical Center/Care Group, Boston, Massachusetts

    c) The Harry R. Horvitz Center for Palliative Medicine, The Cleveland Clinic Foundation, Cleveland, Ohio

    d) Massachusetts General Hospital Palliative Care Hospital, Boston, Massachusetts

    e) Palliative Care Program, Medical College of Virginia Hospitals and Physicians, Virginia Commonwealth University Health System, Richmond, Virginia

    f) Pain and Palliative Care Service, Memorial Sloan-Kettering Cancer Center, New York, New York

    g) The Lilian and Benjamin Hertzberg Palliative Care Institute, Mount Sinai School of Medicine, New York, New York

    h) Palliative Care and Home Hospice Program, Northwestern Memorial Hospital, Chicago, Illinois

    i) Comprehensive Palliative Care Service, University of Pittsburgh, Pittsburgh, Pennsylvania

B. Patient preferences for care at the end of life

1. Two Gallop polls found that 9 out of 10 respondents preferred to be cared for at home if they were terminally ill with less than 6 months left to live[13, 14]

2. In the 1996 Gallop survey 70% of respondents said they would seek hospice care, but 62% indicated that they would still seek curative care.

3. Actual locations of death according to the 1997 Institutes of Medicine Report

    a) 57% of persons die in the hospital (excludes dead on arrival [DOA])

    b) 17% of persons die in nursing homes

    c) 20% of persons die in the home

C.   Reimbursement

1.   Medicare (36–74%)

2.   Medicaid (0–20%)

3.   Private insurance (10–34%)—includes HMO, Blue Shield, Commercial insurances

4.   Indigent Funds (17–20%)

5.   Self-Pay (2–11%)

6.   Medicaid SSI (0–6%)

D.   Funding Sources for research and clinical programs

1.   Federal Grants

2.   Private and public foundations

3.   Industry grants

4.   Endowments and other philanthropic efforts

5.   In-kind support

E.   Organizational structure and admission patterns

1.   Variety of structures

   a)   Two independent academic medical centers merged with a hospital and physician network to form a corporation

   b)   Tertiary center and community hospital merger

   c)   Cancer center

   d)   Private non-profit academic medical center

   e)   Two tertiary teaching hospitals/medical centers

   f)   Private, non-profit group practice with hospitals and family health centers

   g)   Public non-profit hospital

F.   Accreditation

1.   There is currently no mandatory nationwide certification or accreditation for palliative care

2.   JCAHO accreditation for hospitals covers inpatient palliative services

3.   Some palliative care services with hospice components have sought Medicare certification

G.   Patient Information

1.   Diagnoses

   a)   Cancer (53–100%)

   b)   HIV (2–12%)

   c)   Dementia (3–7%)

   d)   Cardiovascular (6–19%)

    e)   End-Stage Disease

        (1)   Lung (3–7%)

        (2)   Liver (5–7%)

        (3)   Renal (1–4%)

    f)   Neurological (0–5%)

    g)   Other (0–5%)

2. Length of Stay (LOS)

    a)   Average LOS range (5 days–71 days)

3. Location of death (regionally dependent on available beds)

    a)   Hospital (6–51%)

    b)   At home (22–68%)

    c)   Nursing home (2–20%)

    d)   Inpatient hospice (11–29%)

    e)   Other (6–29%)

4. Ethnicity

    a)   Black (11–70%)

    b)   White (27–75%)

    c)   Hispanic (1–23%)

    d)   Black Hispanic (1%)

    e)   Asian Indian (2%)

    f)   Asian (1%)

    g)   American Indian (1%)

    h)   Other (1%)

    i)   Unknown (2–7%)

5. Examples of patients who may be appropriate for palliative care rather than hospice care include:

    a)   Those on experimental protocols and/or who are receiving palliative chemotherapy and radiation therapy[15]

    b)   Those individuals who are terminally ill but who are not ready to profess an acceptance of death as an inevitable event[16, 17]

    c)   Those patients who are still receiving active treatment for their incurable illness but who can also benefit from support services[18]

    d)   Children with severe birth defects who will die quickly and often in the hospital[19]

    e)   Those with a life-threatening illness but who are considered to be far from the terminal stage[20]

H. Cost Savings and revenue

1. Goal of Palliative Care Units is to improve quality of care

2. Fiscal argument is secondary to quality of care argument

3. Potential savings for third party payors and for patients/families

   a) Palliative Care Unit (PCU) frees up beds for other patients

   b) Shortened hospital stays

   c) Reduced ancillary costs

   d) Reduces unnecessary tests and procedures

4. Limited data exists on palliative care outcomes (See Economics chapter)

   a) One study[21] found that PCU stay when compared to ICU and non-PCU unit stays, reduced "other" charges (medications, diagnostics) by 74%; charges were reduced overall 66%. (80% of patients had cancer, followed by vascular events, AIDS, organ failure)

      (1) Costs were significantly reduced, especially variation in costs. In many cases, cost/day in the PCU were low enough to be covered by the Medicare hospice per diem

      (2) Both costs and charges were significantly reduced in a case control study

      (3) Patient and family satisfaction was high

      (4) Results indicate that appropriate care given to terminally ill patients in a high volume medical center appears to significantly lower costs

REFERENCES

1. Conner, S.R., *New initiatives transforming hospice care.* The Hospice Journal, 1999. **14**(3/4): p. 193–203.

2. O'Connor, P., *Hospice vs. palliative care.* The Hospice Journal, 1999. **14**(3/4): p. 123–137.

3. Byock, I.R., *Hospice and palliative care: A parting of the ways or a path to the future.* Journal of Palliative Medicine, 1998. **1**: p. 165–76.

4. Portenoy, P.R., *Defining Palliative Care.* 1998, Newsletter, Dept. of Pain and Palliative Care—Beth Israel Medical Center.

5. Brenner, R., *Hospice care and palliative care: A perspective from experience.* The Hospice Journal, 1999. **14**(3/4): p. 155–166.

6. The SUPPORT Principal Investigators, *A controlled trial to improve care for seriously ill patients.* JAMA, 1995. **274**: p. 1591–1598.

7. Matzo, M.L. and D.W. Sherman, *Palliative care nursing: Quality care to the end of life.* 2001, New York: Springer Publishing.

8. National Hospice Organization, *A pathway for patients and families facing terminal illness.* 1997, National Hospice Organization: Arlington, VA. p. 5–6.

9. World Health Organization, *Cancer Pain Relief and Palliative Care.* 1990. 152.

10. Canadian Palliative Care Association, *Palliative care: Towards a consensus in standardized principles of practice.* 1995: Canadian Palliative Care Association.

11. Field, M.J. and C.K. Cassel, *Approaching death: Improving care at the end of life.* 1997, Institute of Medicine Task Force: Washington, DC.

12. Storey, P. and C.F. Knight, *Hospice/palliative care training for physicians (UNIPACS 2, 2, 4, 6).* 1996 & 1997, American Academy of Hospice and Palliative Medicine.

13. Foreman, J., *70% would pick hospice.* The Boston Globe, 1996. **250 (96)**(October 4): p. A3.

14. National Hospice and Palliative Care Organization, *Facts and figures on hospice care in America.* 2001, National Hospice and Palliative Care Organization.

15. Beresford, L., *The questions of growth.* Hospice, 1995. **6(4)**: p. 24–26.

16. Levetown, M., *Different—and needing to be more available.* Hospice, 1995. **6(5)**: p. 15-16, 36.

17. Ewald, R., *Orphaned by AIDS.* Hospice, 1995. **6(5)**: p. 28–32.

18. Clark, D., B. Neale, and P. Heather, *Contracting for palliative care.* Social Sciences and Medicine, 1995. **40**(9): p. 1193–1202.

19. Rogers, B., *When young life is lost.* Hospice, 1995. **6(5)**: p. 24–27.

20. Lewis, L., *Many-party harmony.* Hospice, 1995. **6(5)**: p. 8–9.

21. Payne, S.K., et al., *A high volume specialist palliative care unit (PCU) and team reduces end of life (EOL) costs.* 2001, American Society of Clinical Oncology.

GENERAL REFERENCES

Abu-Saad, H.H. (2000). Palliative care: An international view. *Patient Education and Counseling, 41*: 15–22.

Dush, D.M. (1993). High-tech, aggressive palliative care: In the service of quality of life, *Journal of Palliative Care*, 9(1): 37–41.

Ferrell, B.R. & Coyle, N. (2001). *Textbook of palliative nursing*. Oxford: Oxford University Press.

Saunders, C. (2000). The evolution of palliative care. *Patient Education and Counseling*, 41: 7–13.

Sheehan, D. & Forman, W. (1996). *Hospice and palliative care: Concepts and practice*. Sudbury, MA. Jones and Bartlett, 1–10.

Sherman, D.W. (1999). End of life care: Challenges and opportunities for health care professionals. *The Hospice Journal, 14*(3/4): 109–121.

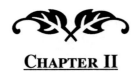

Chapter II

Interdisciplinary Collaborative Practice in the Hospice and Palliative Care Settings

Ellen C. Rooney, RN, C, BSN
Molly Poleto, BSN, RN, CHPN

I. Introduction

Interdisciplinary team (IDT) members represent a variety of disciplines including individuals from medicine, nursing, social work, spiritual, dietary and bereavement counseling, volunteer services, pharmacy and other allied therapies as needed who work together with the patient and family to develop, implement, and evaluate a care plan that addresses the patient and family's needs.

II. Coordinate and Supervise

A. Coordinate patient care with other health providers

1. Incorporate each discipline's assessment of the patient/family into the comprehensive plan of care

2. Facilitate the sharing of patient and family concerns identified by IDT members and incorporate their recommendations for interventions into the ongoing plan of care

3. Establish care goals based on the quality of life needs identified by the patient

4. Identify other healthcare providers (speech therapists and pathologists, physical therapists, occupational therapists, recreation therapists, and others) who will assist in providing comfort, pain and symptom management in the four domains of the patient's quality of life[1]

   a) Physical well-being (control and relief of symptoms and maintenance of function and independence)

   b) Psychological well-being (sense of control in the face of life-threatening illness, emotional distress, altered life priorities, and fears of the unknown)

    c)   Social well-being (roles and relationships)

    d)   Spiritual well-being (ability to maintain hope and derive meaning from the experience)

  5.   Systematically review and routinely update the plan of care to ensure goals defined by the patient and family are being addressed and that continuity of care is being maintained

B.   Supervise unlicensed assistive personnel (UAP)

  1.   Provide an individualized patient care plan for UAP that details a description of the patient's needs and the interventions to be performed

  2.   Provide written instructions regarding communication when a patient care problem arises

  3.   Encourage feedback from UAP about success, observations, or problems of care interventions

  4.   Observe the provision or giving of personal care and the interactions between the patient and family and UAP

  5.   Document on the appropriate form, supervision and teaching of care procedures of UAP

  6.   Provide ongoing support and education

C.   Arrange for medical equipment, supplies and medications

  1.   Assess the need for durable medical equipment (DME) and supplies and obtain orders, if required

  2.   After assessment of the patient's symptoms, and in consultation with the primary physician, obtain orders for medications

  3.   Incorporate into the plan of care any medical equipment, supplies and/or medications determined to be necessary

  4.   Follow guidelines (agency, state, federal, etc.) and reimbursement requirements for obtaining medications, medical equipment, and supplies and documentation of same for hospice recipients

D.   Facilitate and coordinate transfer to a different level of care (LOC) for hospice patients

  1.   Transfer to another level of care is based on the medical and/or social needs of the patient (e.g. uncontrolled or resolved pain)

  2.   Levels of care in Medicare/Medicaid Hospice Program (defined in Chapter IX)

    a)   Routine home care

    b)   Continuous home care

    c)   Inpatient respite care

    d)   General inpatient care

  3.   Change in level of care requires

    a)   Discussion with the patient and family and the Interdisciplinary Team (IDT)

    b)   Changes in the plan of care

    c)   A physician's order (in most cases)

    d)   Documentation in the patient's record

E.   Facilitate and coordinate transfer to a different care setting

1.   Transfer to a different care setting may occur when a patient moves out of the service area covered by a hospice or palliative care provider or when the patient chooses a different hospice or palliative care provider in the same area

2.   Discuss possible change in provider status with primary physician and involve physician in process as warranted

3.   Coordinate transfer with the other hospice/palliative care service in order to maintain continuity of care

4.   Facilitate the patient's adjustment to another setting by collaborating with the IDT members to identify possible problems and stress factors patient and family may experience

5.   Hospice Medicare/Medicaid benefit patients may transfer to a different hospice program only once per benefit period

6.   Discharge from hospice or palliative care is an option that may be chosen by the patient/family in order to receive treatment not covered under the hospice plan of care, to receive care from a different service provider, e.g. skilled nursing facility, non-contracted hospital, or because of dissatisfaction with the service being provided:

    a)   Discuss the change with the primary physician

    b)   If patient is on hospice benefit, provide appropriate release form for patient to sign

7.   Withdrawal from all services (whether hospice or palliative care) may be initiated by patient/family for any reason

    a)   Consider a family conference with the appropriate members of the IDT to review and address concerns of patient and family and to provide information and support to assist in patient/family decision making process

    b)   Discuss change with primary physician; initiate any paperwork necessary for the change

    c)   Initiate required documentation

    d)   Coordinate referrals for provision of on-going health care, i.e., physical therapy, DME vendor, etc.

III. Collaborate

A.   Collaborate with the patient's primary physician who will:

1.   Oversee the medical aspects of the patient's plan of care

2.   Assure medical eligibility for healthcare services, i.e., hospice benefit, palliative care service, skilled nursing facility

3.   Provide information regarding medical conditions including those unrelated to the terminal illness

4.   Participate in the initial development of plan of care

5.   Provide ongoing medical management and orders for medications, treatments, symptom management interventions, level of care transfers, and changes in care settings

B.   Participate in the development of an individualized interdisciplinary plan of care for the patient and family

1.   Develop a plan of care with the IDT, which begins prior to admission, and follows through to the end of life (or discharge from the program for other reasons), and into bereavement care for the family

2.   Individualize the plan in accordance with the expressed needs of the patient and family for achieving and/or maintaining quality of life as defined by them

3.   Recognize that the plan of care is continually evaluated and updated to meet ongoing and changing patient and family needs

C.   Demonstrate awareness of techniques of conflict resolution[2]

1.   Levels of Conflict

a)   Intrapersonal—within the individual

b)   Interpersonal—between two individuals

c)   Intra-organizational—within the organization

d)   Inter-organizational—between two organizations

2.   Factors that may lead to conflict

a)   Ambiguous role boundaries, roles that are changing, protective territorialism of role area

b)   Interdisciplinary professional rivalry

c)   Communication barriers; small problems that are not addressed due to of lack of time, opportunity, or ability

d)   Leadership style that is not appropriate for the situation, or congruent with the needs of the team

e)   Decision making that may exclude input from individuals involved

f)   Team members with differing goals and expectations

g)   Prior conflicts, displaced hostility

h)   Differing personality styles

i)   Continuing change; change threatening the existence of individual positions or the program; change which affects team members unequally

j)   Scarcity of resources

3.   Techniques for mediation of conflict

a)   Listen with understanding and not evaluation

b)   Develop ground rules and procedures

    c)   Identify the issues

    d)   Clarify the nature of the problems seen by both sides

    e)   Bring conflict into the open, use it as potential for change

    f)   Reduce the area of conflict. Both sides listen to problems and agree to work only on those problems listed by both sides

    g)   Identify short and long term goals

    h)   Create and evaluate as many solutions as possible

    i)   Agree on one solution, record it as an agreement

    j)   Plan implementation and subsequent re-evaluation

D. Utilize techniques of effective group process

1. Coordination and continuity of care are accomplished, in part, by assurance that the plan of care is implemented by each team member responsible for patient and family care

2. Collaboration is accomplished by open, respectful, forthright communication with team members, by ongoing discussion of the care goals in all care settings, and by addressing conflict among team members regarding patient and family care

3. Conflict may result when role blurring occurs

    a)   Recognize that blurring of roles is a *normal* byproduct of shared responsibilities for care of patient and family

    b)   Recognize the individuality of team members who will incorporate various techniques and approaches in their practice

    c)   Recognize that conflict can be uncomfortable, and provide support to individual members and the team as a whole

    d)   Evaluate outcomes of conflict management support, e.g., fewer negative interactions among team members, fewer complaints about colleague behaviors, and improved collaboration and problem solving

E. Continuously evaluate progression of disease process to verify appropriateness for hospice or palliative care

1. Discuss the trajectory of the disease with the physician and IDT

2. Assess the effectiveness of symptom management interventions that are being implemented to promote comfort

3. Document patient condition and response to interventions in detail sufficient to "paint a picture" of patient status

4. Review with team members the care being provided to ensure that it is appropriate to the stage of the illness

5. Include the patient and family in the evaluation process

6. Discuss each team member's role in providing support and education about life-extending therapies for the patient, if requested, keeping in mind the patient's and family's goals

F.   Encourage family participation in IDT decisions

1.   Patient and family are considered the unit of care; the family needs to be fully involved when the patient is receiving hospice or palliative care services and may need guidance and support in identifying mutual goals

2.   The IDT develops the overall plan of care in collaboration with the patient and family, to provide coordinated care which emphasizes supportive services such as home care, pain and symptom management and inpatient services, information concerning financial issues, safety issues, and concerns with cultural practices

3.   Patients and families who participate in the decision making process retain a higher degree of autonomy in their lives; the transition through the later phases of the disease process and into the dying stages is enhanced by such participation

IV. Advocate

A.   Act as a patient and family advocate with other team members

B.   Educate patient and family caregivers about the "benefits and burdens" of treatments and provide support for their preferences and needs

C.   Act as a resource for hospice and palliative care within different care settings

D.   Know the patient care setting policies and procedures for advanced directives, medical orders, changes in levels of care, etc., and share this information with the IDT

V.   Practice Issues

A.   Identify and incorporate standards into practice

1.   Hospice and Palliative Nurses Association standards reflect the current status of nursing within the field and guides competent clinical care through continued evaluation

a)   *Standards of Hospice Nursing Practice* (Appendix 4)

b)   *Standards of Professional Performance* (Appendix 4)

2.   Other Standards that impact the delivery of nursing care in hospice and palliative care include:

a)   National Hospice and Palliative Care Organization's Standards of Practice for Hospice Programs[3]

b)   JCAHO Standards

c)   Community Health Accreditation Program (CHAP) Standards

d)   Accreditation Commission for Home Care (ACHC) Standards

e)   ANA Standards of clinical nursing practice

f)   State Nurse Practice Act

B.   Identify and incorporate guidelines into practice

1.   Clinical Practice Guidelines "Management of Cancer Pain"—Agency for Healthcare Research and Quality (AHRQ) (formerly Agency for Health Care Policy and Research [AHCPR])

2.   World Health Organization—3 Step Analgesic Ladder (under revision as of 2002)

3.   National Hospice and Palliative Care Organization

    a)   Medical Guidelines for Determining Prognosis in Selected Non-Cancer Diseases[4]

    b)   Standards of Practice for Hospice Programs[3]

    c)   NHPCO Guidelines for Nursing in Hospice Care

    d)   Symptom Management Algorithms: A Handbook for Palliative Care[5]

C.   Identify and incorporate legal regulations into practice

1.   Medicare Conditions of Participation—Centers for Medicare & Medicaid Services (CMS) (Formerly known as HCFA)

2.   OSHA regulations

3.   Medicaid regulations (where applicable)

4.   CMS Long Term Care regulations

D.   Education of the public on end-of-life issues

1.   Advance Directives

    a)   Patient Self Determination Act of 1991 assured the right to accept or refuse treatment under state laws[6]

    b)   Each state incorporates its Advance Directives in its state legal code (definition and codes will vary from state to state)

    c)   Methods of executing advance directives

        (1)   Living Will: a document that communicates the patient's wishes about end of life treatment should he or she become incapacitated

        (2)   Durable Power of Attorney for Health Care (also known as "Health Care Proxy" or "Health Care Agent"): a legal document that authorizes another person to make health care decisions for the patient should he or she become unable to do so

        (3)   "Five Wishes": a questionnaire that guides people in making essential decisions about care at the end of their life; this advance directive is legally valid in 34 states and the District of Columbia (the other 16 require a specific state-mandated form)

    d)   The hospice or palliative care service should counsel patient/families to complete advance directives and,

        (1)   Obtain copies of the patient's advance directives

        (2)   Advance directives should be completed/recorded according to state and federal regulations

2.   Termination of treatment—competent patients have the right to determine the nature and duration of treatment

3.   Do not resuscitate orders (DNR)

a)   All IDT members should review and be familiar with state laws regarding resuscitation procedures in all care settings

b)   Do not resuscitate (DNR) orders are a written legal document signed by the physician

c)   Generally, unless there is a physician order to the contrary, the patient must be resuscitated if pulmonary and/or cardiac functions cease; this is a general standard of care in the United States

d)   DNR orders are not required for admission to a hospice or palliative care service

e)   It is recommended that hospice programs have policies that inform the patient and family that the hospice is not financially responsible for procedures, e.g., resuscitation, curative treatments, that are not part of the plan of care

f)   DNR orders may be verbally revoked by the patient at any time and *sometimes* by the family on behalf of the patient; this also varies widely according to state law

g)   Prehospital/outpatient DNR orders are recognized by 38 states

h)   DNR orders are being replaced by "Limitations of Life Sustaining Treatments"

4.   Patient Bill of Rights

a)   Rights and responsibilities as established by Medicare, JCAHO, CHAP, and state licensing regulations (where applicable)

b)   Establish a confidential complaint procedure in policy and procedures that can be implemented for patient and family complaints

E.   **Participate in evaluating and providing educational materials for patients and families**

1.   Materials and information provided in various formats (verbal, written, videotape, audiotape, electronic media)

2.   Assess for appropriate reading level to ensure comprehension

F.   **Access educational resources from multimedia sources**

1.   Conference videos

2.   Video tapes

3.   Internet resources—see Appendix 2

G.   **Utilize research to improve quality of care outcomes and quality of life for patient/family and the public at large**

1.   Reasons to plan, implement and apply hospice and palliative care nursing research

a)   To develop, refine, and extend the scientific base of knowledge

b)   To be professionally accountable to patients and families and the general public

c)   To improve end of life care for patients and families in all practice settings

d)   To enhance the art and science of and to define the parameters of palliative and hospice nursing care

e)   To define the distinct and unique roles of palliative care and hospice in the delivery of health care

f)   To document the social relevancy and efficacy of hospice and palliative care practice to others

g)   To justify the allocation of financial resources to hospice and palliative care services by providing data regarding cost effectiveness

H.   **Educate health care providers regarding the hospice benefits under Medicare/Medicaid.** (See Chapter X: Economic Issues in Hospice and Palliative Care for a description of the Medicare Hospice Benefit)

I.   **Participate in Quality Improvement, an ongoing and proactive process that:**

1.   Identifies system problems and deficiencies

2.   Identifies processes that continually improve care outcomes

3.   Establishes new ways of providing high quality, cost-effective care

VI. Professional Development

A.   **Contribute to the professional development of peers, colleagues and others as preceptor, educator, or mentor**

1.   Mentor student nurses, social worker and chaplain interns, medical students and others

2.   Precept new staff and provide guidance and support

3.   Provide educational forums

4.   Network with peers to share information and promote connectedness within the profession

5.   Serve as consultant to other providers

6.   Assist in the development and evaluation of preceptor/mentor programs

B.   **Identify strategies to resolve ethical concerns related to end-of-life care**

1.   Ethical principles[7]

    a)   *Autonomy:* A form of personal liberty. The individual determines his or her own course and plan of action; self determination

    b)   *Veracity:* To tell the truth and not deceive others: as in informed consent; providing enough information in order to make an informed decision

    c)   *Beneficence:* duty to help others; prevent or remove harm; balance of help and harm; to do good

   d)   *Nonmaleficence:* avoiding intentional infliction of harm; to do no harm

   e)   *Justice:* "equals ought to be treated equally"[7]; giving what is due or owed; distributing resources fairly

2.   Ethical dilemma: A situation involving a choice between equally unsatisfactory alternatives, for example:

   a)   Violating confidentiality: Is it ever acceptable to violate patient confidentiality?

      (1)   Dilemma: Patient's right to autonomy vs. the professional's duty to protect patients from themselves

      (2)   Example: Patient's expression of suicidal ideation or for assisted suicide

   b)   Telling the truth: Is it ever acceptable *not* to tell a terminally ill person he or she is dying?

      (1)   Dilemma: Professional's duty to the patient vs. duty to the family

      (2)   Example: Family does not want patient to be told the prognosis

3.   HPNA *Standard of Professional Performance V.* **Ethics:** The hospice [and palliative] nurse's decisions and actions on behalf of patient and family are determined in an ethical manner[8]

   a)   The hospice nurse's practice is guided by the current ANA Code for Nurses and other professional statements of the profession

   b)   The hospice nurse maintains and protects confidentiality

   c)   The hospice nurse acts as a patient and family advocate

   d)   The hospice nurse delivers care in a nonjudgmental and nondiscriminatory manner that is sensitive to patient and family diversity

   e)   The hospice nurse delivers care in a manner that preserves/protects patient and family autonomy, dignity, and rights

   f)   The hospice nurse collaborates with the interdisciplinary team and seeks other available resources to help in the formulation of ethical decisions

   g)   The hospice nurse recognizes his/her own values and beliefs when assisting in the formulation of ethical decisions

   h)   The hospice nurse maintains and updates her/his knowledge of ethical issues

   i)   The hospice nurse recognizes and accepts a fiduciary relationship with the patient and family, including the recognition and maintenance of professional boundaries

4.   Ethical decision-making process (can be employed by individuals and teams)

   a)   Identify and clarify the issue, including interested parties

   b)   Identify the values that interested parties use in addressing this issue

   c)   Gather information

   d)   Determine the ethical principle(s) and theories involved

   e)   Identify the possible risks and benefits of all alternatives

  f) Discuss alternatives with other individuals and team as appropriate, working together to build consensus

  g) Make a decision

C. Participate in peer review

D. Maintain professional boundaries between patients/family and staff

 1. Understand team member roles

 2. Maintaining boundaries minimizes conflict

 3. Work within defined role limits as appropriate, but be flexible, able, and willing to blend roles when necessary

 4. Each team member should be aware of need to set limits/boundaries for self and others when interacting with patients and families

 5. Foster independence of patients and families; empower them to maintain maximum control of their lives

E. Participate in professional self-care (e.g., stress management)

 1. Accept that stress exists and will be experienced by everyone who works with the dying and their families

 2. Acknowledge that people often do not recognize stress in themselves

 3. Be aware that clinical competency helps to reduce stress—take advantage of educational opportunities

 4. Increase knowledge regarding end of life care, bereavement support and public policy affecting end of life care

 5. Develop and maintain strong personal support systems

 6. Practice spiritual self-care

 7. Set reasonable and attainable goals

 8. Maintain a balance in interactions with patients and families. Self-awareness is important in maintenance of appropriate boundaries.

 9. Secure a sense of closure after patients' deaths.

 10. Get adequate rest, eat a proper diet and participate in regular physical exercise

 11. Remain involved with the team for mutual support and a feeling of belonging

F. Promote utilization, development, and implementation of research in a variety of settings

 1. Participate in research activities (see Practice Issues—Section V)

 2. Critical steps in research

  a) Develop an idea

  b) Define the problem/issue/question

  c) Collect background information

    d)   Develop a written plan

    e)   State objectives or hypothesis

    f)   Determine research design

    g)   Collect data

    h)   Analyze data

    i)   Draw conclusions

    j)   Apply findings to clinical practice as appropriate

    k)   Disseminate findings to colleagues

G.   Read medical and nursing journals to remain current in knowledge of treatment options and end of life care

H.   Participate in professional nursing organization activities

1.   Hospice and Palliative Nurses Association

    a.   National

    b.   Regional

2.   State organizations

3.   American Nurses Association

4.   Attend state and national conferences

5.   Obtain certification in specialty areas of practice, i.e. hospice and palliative nursing

I.   Maintain personal continuing education plan to update knowledge

1.   Track attendance at conferences and meetings

2.   List educational opportunities by title and presenter

3.   Retain copies of handouts and number of hours attended

J.   Advocate for the profession

1.   Keep informed about the state and federal policies that impact end-of-life care

2.   Know and support various professional organizations' positions on end-of-life care; maintain open dialogue on this topic

3.   Educate policy makers, legislators about the needs of families experiencing end-of-life care

REFERENCES

1.   Grant, M., *Introduction: Nausea and vomiting, quality of life and the oncology nurse.* Oncology Nursing Forum, 1997. **24**(Supp 7): p. 5–7.

2.   Weiss, D.H., *Conflict resolution.* 1998, New York: AMACOM.

3.   National Hospice and Palliative Care Organization, *Standards of Practice for Hospice Programs.* 2000, Alexandria, VA: National Hospice and Palliative Care Organization.

4.   National Hospice Organization, *Medical guidelines for determining prognosis in selected non-cancer diseases.* 2nd Edition ed. 1996, Arlington, VA: National Hospice Organization.

5.   Wrede-Seaman, L., *Symptom management algorithms: A handbook for palliative care.* 2nd Edition ed. 1999, Yakima, WA: Intellicard.

6.   House of Representatives, *Omnibus Reconciliation Act of 1990.* 1990.

7.   Beauchamp, J.L. and J.F. Childress, *Principles of BioMedical Ethics.* 4th ed. 1994, New York: Oxford University Press.

8.   Hospice Nurses Association Standards and Accreditation Committee, *Standards of hospice nursing practice and professional performance.* 1995, Pittsburgh, PA: Hospice Nurses Association.

GENERAL REFERENCES

American Nurses Association. (1991). *Promotion of comfort and relief of pain in dying patients.* (Position statement). Washington, DC: Author.

American Nurses Association.   (1994). *Assisted suicide.* (Position statement). Washington, DC: Author.

Coyle, N. (2001). Introduction to palliative nursing. In B.R. Ferrell & N. Coyle (Eds.). *Textbook of palliative nursing* (pp. 3–6). New York: Oxford University Press.

Dodge, C. (2000). Health care without borders: The interdisciplinary approach. *Geriatric Times, 1*(1). Retrieved October 11, 2001, from http://www.medinfosource.com/gt/g000604.html

Egan, K.A. & Labyak, M.J. (2001). Hospice care: A model for quality end-of-life care. In B.R. Ferrell & N. Coyle (Eds.). *Textbook of palliative nursing* (pp. 7–26). New York: Oxford University Press.

Hunter, W.R.. (2001). Hospice and palliative medicine: Irreconcilable differences...or destined for the altar? *The Hospice Professional, 1, (1)*, pp. 1–6.

Lattanzi-Licht, M., Mahoney, J.J. & Miller, G.W. (1998). *The hospice choice: In pursuit of a peaceful death.* New York: Simon & Schuster.

Lynn, J. & Harold J. (1999). *Handbook for mortals: Guidance for people facing serious illnesses.* New York: Oxford University Press.

Oncology Nursing Society. (1992). *Cancer and aging: The mandate for oncology nursing* (Position statement). Pittsburgh: Author.

Oncology Nursing Society. (1998). *Oncology Nursing Society and the Association of Oncology Social Work joint position on end-of-life care.* (Position Statement). Pittsburgh, PA: Author.

Scanlon, C. (2001). Public policy and end-of-life care: The nurse's role. In B.R. Ferrell & N. Coyle (Eds.). *Textbook of palliative nursing* (pp. 682–689). New York: Oxford University Press.

The American Society of Pain Management Nurses. (1998). *End-of-life care.* (Position Statement) Pensacola, FL: Author.

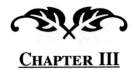

CHAPTER III

PATTERNS OF DISEASE PROGRESSION

Connie Dahlin, MSN, RN, CHPN
Kathy Kalina, RN, BSN

I.   **HIV/AIDS (Human Immunodeficiency Virus)/(Acquired Immunodeficiency Disease Syndrome)**

A.   **Cumulative Number of AIDS cases**

1.   US—753,907 persons with the disease

2.   Worldwide 36.1 million persons estimated with the disease

3.   Total Deaths

a)   US—438,795 persons have died from AIDS

b)   Worldwide—21.8 million deaths

c)   Largest number is males from ages 30–45

B.   **Definition: AIDS is characterized by infections and cancers that are the consequence of extreme immunodeficiency caused by infection with the human immunodeficiency virus (HIV). AIDS is the most advanced stage of HIV infection. HIV is a retrovirus that attaches to a cell and enters it.**

C.   **Transmission occurs from:**

1.   Sexual Contact—rectal, vaginal, and more rarely, oral contact with an infected person

2.   Contaminated blood products

3.   Contaminated needles shared by intravenous drug users

4.   Organ transplant and insemination from infected donors

5.   Prenatal and perinatal exposure for newborns (pregnancy, childbirth, and breastfeeding)

6.   Occupational injuries (e.g., needle sticks, sharps)

D.   Pathogenesis

1.   HIV infection with progression to AIDS

2.   Virus attaches to T lymphocytes and macrophages facilitated by cytokine receptors

3.   Uncoating of the virus

4.   Conversion of viral RNA to proviral DNA by reverse transcriptase

5.   Proviral DNA incorporated into the cell nucleus

6.   Transcription of DNA into RNA

7.   RNA expression and formation of infectious virion translates cell into proteins and enzymes

E.   Disease Progression

1.   Primary or Acute Infection

    a)   Occurs when virus enters the body and replicates in the blood and lymphatics

    b)   Initial decrease of T cells

    c)   Viral load increases

    d)   Within 5–30 days of exposure, flu-like symptoms characteristic of infection include fever, sore throat, skin rash, and lymphadenopathy, and myalgia

    e)   Seroconversion usually within 6–12 weeks

2.   Clinical Latency

    a)   Chronic, asymptomatic state where clinically stable

    b)   Resolution of flu-like symptoms

    c)   Virus continues to replicate, most likely at some individually defined set point or rate

3.   Early Symptomatic Stage

    a)   Often occurs after years of infection

    b)   CD4 counts drops below 500 cells/mm^3

    c)   HIV viral load increases

4.   Late Symptomatic Stage

    a)   CD4 counts drop below 200 cells/mm^3

    b)   HIV viral load increases above 100,000/ml

    c)   Opportunistic infections occur including

        (1)   PCP

        (2)   HIV encephalopathy

        (3)   HIV wasting

        (4)   TB

        (5)   Bacterial infections

      (6)   Oral/Fungal candidiasis

      (7)   AIDS related malignancies

          (a)   Kaposi's Sarcoma

          (b)   Non-Hodgkin's Lymphoma

          (c)   Invasive Cervical/Anal Cancer

   5.   Advanced HIV Disease

      a)   CD4 counts drop below 50 cells/mm^3

      b)   Immune system severely impaired

      c)   Further AIDS related infections/diagnoses

      d)   Pneumonia-Pneumocystis Carinii, Mycobacterium Tuberculosis

      e)   Skin Lesions—Kaposi's Sarcoma, Herpes simplex, Mollusum Contagiosum, Scabies

      f)   Psychological—anxiety, depression, isolation

      g)   Neurological—dementia, meningitis, toxoplasmosis

      h)   CMV Retinitis

      i)   Fatigue

      j)   Poor functional status

      k)   Wasting syndrome

      l)   Pain

      m)   GI—diarrhea, anal and perirectal lesions, incontinence

F.   Issues in Progressive Illness

   1.   The "roller coaster" unpredictable nature of the disease and its progression

   2.   The treatable nature of the opportunistic infections

   3.   Uncertainty of prognosis

   4.   Availability of new conventional and non-traditional treatments

   5.   AIDS is more a "chronic" and less a "terminal" disease

   6.   When/if to discontinue treatment: often it remains appropriate to continue Gancyclovir (for CMV retinitis/blindness prevention) and some other antiretrovirals and opportunistic infection prophylaxis until the final stages of the illness

   7.   Death not from HIV/AIDS itself, but from complications caused by it

G.   Potential Care Differences in the person with HIV/AIDS

   1.   Non-traditional lifestyles and values

   2.   Alternative family structures

   3.   Large network for consumer advocacy and education about treatment and support

4. Youth of most patients

5. Multiple losses within the community

H. Hospice and palliative care program issues

1. Financial concerns regarding available treatments and medications

2. Need for staff education regarding unique care issues and fears arising from stigma of diseases and ignorance

3. Inflexibility of hospice admission criteria

4. When does a change from palliative care outside of a hospice framework to palliative care within a hospice framework become appropriate?

I. Special grief issues in AIDS bereavement

1. For family of origin, friends, and professional caregivers—lack of recognition in care giving process. Result may be increased expressions of rage, fear, shame, guilt, helplessness, physical symptoms, self-destructiveness, insecurity, numbness and cynicism

2. Disenfranchised grief

3. Homophobia and heterosexism

4. Stigma of substance abuse

5. Stigma of AIDS and HIV leads to secrecy and isolation

6. Guilt of survivors

7. The feelings, fears related to the illness itself, complications, and uncertainty regarding the course of the disease

8. Multiple and continuing losses

J. Treatment

1. Therapy recommended for all patients with primary HIV infections and symptomatic individuals

2. Immune therapy: research continues but the high mutation rate of the virus and the incorporation of the virus into the host cell nucleic acid, makes the development of immune therapy challenging and difficult

3. Antiviral therapy: Antiretroviral drugs, protease inhibitors, nucleoside reverse-transcriptase inhibitors, non-nucleoside reverse-transcriptase inhibitors

K. Other symptom management issues particular to AIDS

1. AIDS-related diarrhea

   a) One of the most common symptoms seen in AIDS patients; contributes significantly to morbidity and cachexia and wasting syndrome

   b) Small bowel—profuse, non-bloody, related to food intake

   c) Large bowel—frequent, small, mucoid, bloody, LLQ cramps, tenesmus, less related to food intake

    d)   Causes—cryptosporidium (protozoal infection) is the cause in 1 of 3 cases; other causes include salmonella, shigella, campylobacter, clostridium difficile, and giardia

    e)   Treatment—treat the cause; use bulk forming agents; Lomotil®, Imodium®, octreotide (Sandostatin®)

2.   Pain

    a)   Peripheral neuropathies are common

    b)   Rectal pain should be considered due to herpes until proven otherwise; squamous cell carcinoma of the anus is a very treatable cancer seen in these patients

    c)   Headache from opportunistic infections also common

    d)   Dysphagia—pain in the mouth or throat that causes difficulty in swallowing; usually related to fungal infections, herpes simplex, T-cell Lymphomas or Kaposi's Sarcoma; treat the underlying cause and provide symptomatic support

    e)   Dermatologic problems—psoriasis, rashes and dry skin are common

    f)   Cardiac disease—an infrequent clinical problem in HIV, but abnormalities have been found on a majority of patients either upon autopsy or invasive exploration; as persons with AIDS live longer, symptoms related to myocarditis and cardiomyopathy may appear. In addition, lipid and other metabolic abnormalities related to anti-retrovirals therapy may affect development of CAD.

AIDS-RELATED CONDITIONS*

General Information

Condition	Signs and Symptoms	Treatments[1]
Opportunistic Infections		
		(Note: meds ending in "zole" treat fungal infections)
Fungal:		
• Aspergillus	Rare; usually seen in end stage disease; cough, elevated LDH, fever, pleuritic chest pain	(Amphotericin-B, Itraconazole
• Candida	Often first opportunistic infection, can occur in (mouth, esophagus, vagina, rectum, skin), white, furry or cheesy patches on mucous membranes with burning pain and dysphagia, loss of appetite, vaginal or rectal burning, itching, & discharge	Nystatin, Fluconazole, Chlortrimazole, Miconazole Amphotericin-B
• Coccidiodomycosis	Lung primary site of infection, may affect skin meninges, lymph nodes, liver; cough, fatigue, fever, malaise, pleuritic chest pain, weight loss	Amphotericin-B, Fluconazole,

---

* Prepared by Susan Corrado, RN, CRNH, HospiceCare Inc., Madison, WI., 1996; Reviewed and revised, 2001.

General Information

Condition	Signs and Symptoms	Treatments[1]
• Cryptococcus Meningitis	Malaise, nausea, fatigue, behavior changes, headache, memory loss, mental status changes, photophobia, occasionally pneumonia	Amphotericin-B Fluconazole
• Histoplasmosis	Begins in lungs, may become systemic; lymphadenopathy, fever, cough, anemia, leukopenia, thrombocytopenia, hepatosplenomegaly, malaise, weight loss, skin lesions, dyspnea, anemia	Amphotericin-B, Itraconazole or Fluconazole

Bacterial:

Condition	Signs and Symptoms	Treatments[1]
• MAI/MAC (Mycobacterium Avium Complex)	Occurs late in HIV infection, approx. 50% incidence; fever, weight loss, fatigue, diarrhea, anorexia, thrombocytopenia, hepatospleno-megaly, night sweats, abdominal pain, weakness, dizziness, palpable abdominal lymphadenopathy	Macrolide, (Clarithromycin or Azithromycin), & Rifabutin, & Ethambutol for acute treatment Prophylaxis with Rifabutin or Clarithromycin or Ethambutol _(Combination treatment is most effective; rx & condition similar to TB)_
• Nocardiosis	Causes liquefaction, necrosis, abscesses, common in lung and CNS, may affect abdomen; _lung:_ fever, malaise, night sweats, productive cough, weight loss; _CNS:_ brain abscesses; _abdomen:_ abdominal pain and tenderness, ascites, fever	TMP Sulfa
• Salmonellosis	Incidence in patients with AIDS is 100 times greater than in the general population, usual cause is ingestion of contaminated food or direct fecal oral spread; anorexia, chills, diarrhea, fever, sweats, weight loss	Ampicillin or Fluoroquinolone or Ceftriaxone or Cipro or TMP Sulfa for acute treatment. TMP Sulfa or Amoxicillin for maintenance. Consider Rifampin for synergistic effects

General Information

Condition	Signs and Symptoms	Treatments[1]
• Tuberculosis	May be first sign of immunocompromise, multi-drug resistance, approx. 75% have disease outside lung (pleura, lymph nodes, bone marrow, peripheral blood, GI and GU tract, brain, bone, skin, soft tissue, pericardium; cough, hemoptysis, night sweats, weight loss, fever	Isoniazid, Rifampin, Pyrazinamide, & Streptomycin or Ethambutol. Prophylaxis with Isoniazid or Rifampin for those without current active TB

Protozoal
(parasitic infections):

Condition	Signs and Symptoms	Treatments[1]
• Cryptosporidium	Nausea, vomiting, fever, severe watery diarrhea, flatulence, malaise, myalgias, abdominal cramping, weakness, weight loss	Restore immune system with HAART. No currently approved specific agent. Try Paromomycin or nitrazoxanide
• Isosporiasis	Biliary tract obstruction, intractable diarrhea, malabsorption, malnutrition, weakness, weight loss	TMP Sulfa or Pyrimethamine for acute treatment
• PCP (Pneumocystis carinii)	Most common opportunistic infection in persons with HIV, >65% develop PCP; cough, diarrhea, malaise, rales, wheezes, tachypnea, fever, dry cough, weight loss, night sweats, fatigue, dyspnea, weakness	TMP Sulfa or Dapsone as first line drugs. Pentamidine or Clindamycin *as secondary drugs TMP Sulfa (often taken as a prophylactic; reduces incidence by 90%)*
• Toxoplasmosis	Cats and birds often serve as reservoirs for the organism, most common cause of focal encephalitis in patients with AIDS; lethargy, confusion, delusions, paralysis, sensory deficits, focal neurologic deficits, seizures, headache, fever, coma (can cause symptoms in lung, heart and eyes)	Pyrimethamine & Folinic Acid to treat acute infection Second line treatment with Clindamycin or Atovaquone or Clarithromycin or Azithromycin. TMP Sulfa for prophylaxis in those with CD4 < 100/mm^3

General Information

Condition	Signs and Symptoms	Treatments[1]
Viral: • CMV (Cytomegaloviris) colitis	Can be sexually transmitted, latent virus in general population, CMV most common with CD4 counts < 50; weight loss, fatigue, diarrhea (often bloody), cramps, diffuse mucosal ulceration, erythema, esophagitis, gastritis, submucosal hemorrhage	High dose treatment with Ganciclovir or Foscarnet. Life-long daily maintenance with one of the two medications
• CMV (Cytomegaloviris) retinitis	Can be sexually transmitted, latent virus in general population, CMV most common with CD4 counts < 50; blurred vision, perivascular exudate, retinal hemorrhages, scotoma, loss of vision, unilateral visual field loss	Ganciclovir Foscarnet
• Herpes Simplex	Common sexually transmitted disease, disseminated HSV infection can be life-threatening; _general:_ pain, painful vesicular eruption, ulcers; _genital lesions:_ adenopathy, dysuria, lesions in genital area; _orolabial lesions:_ adenopathy, vesicular eruptions on lips, tongue, and oral mucosa; _rectal lesions:_ painful, invasive lesions	Acyclovir
• Herpes Zoster	Caused by reactivation of the virus in dorsal root ganglia, may be first sign of immuno-compromise; itching, deep, aching pain, red rash to vesicles, fatigue, headache, malaise, vesicular rash confined to one dermatome.	Acyclovir or Famciclovir or Ganciclovir or Foscarnet; pain management
• Molluscum Contagiosum	Cutaneous poxvirus infection, sexually transmitted; flesh-colored umbilicated papules along face, neck, scalp, and trunk	Removal, Retin-A
• PML (progressive multifocal leuko-encephalopathy)	Progressive weakness, abnormal gait, ataxia, focal neurological deficits, speech problems, dementia, forgetfulness, incontinence	Experimental treatments only

General Information

Condition	Signs and Symptoms	Treatments[1]
Common Cancers		
• Kaposi's Sarcoma	Cause (Sherman, 2001) symptoms dependent on organ system affected; pigmented purple, red or brownish lesions on skin, in gastrointestinal tract, lung;	Small lesions treated only if painful or causing cosmetic problems; KS lesions highly sensitive to radiation therapy Isolated lesions can be treated with cryotherapy or laser surgery. Interferon alpha with antiretroviral agents may help, as well as single agent or combination chemotherapy
• CNS Lymphoma	One of first malignancies associated with HIV; aphasia, confusion, cranial nerve palsy, headache, hemiparesis, lethargy, memory loss, seizures	Radiation therapy, usually whole brain
• Non-Hodgkin's Lymphoma	Incidence 10%; anorectal abscess, fever, lymphadenopathy, night sweats, weight loss	Chemotherapy, antiretroviral agents may enhance clinical response to chemotherapy
Other Conditions		
• HIV-associated dementia (also called AIDS dementia complex (ADC)	Most common CNS complication in patients with AIDS; *early S & S*: apathy, reduced spontaneity, social withdrawal, agitation, confusion, hallucinations, short term memory loss, (long term memory usually preserved), ataxia, leg weakness, tremors, decreased coordination, impaired handwriting; *late S & S*: global dementia, confusion, delayed verbal responses, vacant stare, restlessness, disinhibition, organic psychosis, motor slowing, truncal ataxia, leg weakness greater than arm weakness; long term prognosis is poor with death following a vegetative state within weeks or months	Zidovudine; palliative management
• Wasting syndrome	Weight loss greater than 10% of usual weight in ≤6 months, chronic diarrhea, chronic weakness, anorexia and fever in the absence of other conditions which cause similar symptoms	Management of symptoms, nutritional counseling and emotional issues related to body image; appetite stimulation may also be tried

II. Neoplastic Conditions

A. Pathophysiology

1. Cancer is a mass of abnormal cells characterized by dysplasia (dissimilar growth), hyperplasia (increased number of cells). The basic features of the cells include:

    a) Unregulated cell growth

    b) Poor cell differentiation

    c) Ability of cells to invade other tissues

    d) Ability to initiate new growth at distant sites

    e) Ability to evade immune system

2. Cancer is second leading cause of death.

    a) The American Cancer Society estimates that over 1.5 million new cases of cancer are diagnosed each year

    b) Approximately 500,000 deaths annually

    c) Since 1990, 16 million new cancer diagnoses[2]

B. Patterns of disease progression

1. Metastatic Process

    a) Angiogenesis—the generation of blood vessels around the primary tumor that increases the chance for tumor cells to reach the bloodstream and ultimately colonize into secondary sites

    b) Attachment or adhesion—tumor cells need to attach themselves to other cells and/or cell matrix proteins

    c) Invasion—tumor cells move across the normal barriers imposed by extracellular matrix

    d) Tumor cell proliferation—a new colony of tumor cells is stimulated to grow at the secondary site

2. Patterns historically predicted by basis of the pattern of lymphatic and venous drainage in the area surrounding the tumor.

C. The signs and symptoms of advanced cancer may include:

1. Asthenia defined as debility, loss of strength, weakness

2. Anorexia and accompanying weight loss and cachexia

3. Pain

4. Nausea

5. Constipation/obstipation

6. Sedation or confusion

7. Dyspnea

8. Edema/swelling

9. Bleeding

10. Infections

D. Treatment Modalities

1. Surgery

a) Removal of tissue to treat cancer locally

b) Prophylactic—Excision, Laser, or cryotherapy to prevent cancer such as for polyps or breast cancer or cervical cancer

c) Diagnostic—obtain tissue to confirm the diagnosis and identify the specific type of cancer (e.g. incisional, excisional, and needle biopsies)

d) Staging—determine the extent of disease

e) Definitive or Curative—curative procedure to remove all of the malignant tumor and a margin of surrounding tissue or removal of tissues to decrease the risk of cancer development, progression, or recurrence

f) Palliative—prolongs life, promotes comfort and quality of life without the goal of curing the illness (e.g. bone stabilization, relief of obstruction, treatment for oncologic emergency, pain management, tumor debulking)

g) Adjuvant or Supportive—surgery is used with other treatment modalities to assess response to treatment or improve cosmetic, and/or functional outcomes (e.g. gastrostomy tube, venous access devices, radioactive implants, implantable pumps)

h) Reconstructive or Rehabilitative—Minimize deformity and improve quality of life

2. Radiation Therapy

a) The use of high-energy radiation (particles or waves) to eradicate cancer cells in local treatment

(1) Delivered by either external beam, referred to as teletherapy (where the source of the ionizing radiation is outside the body)

(2) Internal radiation, referred to as brachytherapy (where the radioactive source in placed directly into a body cavity or directly on the body)

b) Primary therapy—radiation given to eradicate disease

c) Combined modality therapy—

(1) Decrease the risk of local recurrence, in conjunction with surgery and chemotherapy

(2) Increase tumor destruction, in conjunction with chemotherapy

d) Prophylaxis—radiation is used to treat tissues or organs before the disease is clinically evident, as with central nervous system prophylaxis

e) Palliative therapy

(1) Radiation therapy is used to relieve symptoms in patients with advanced disease, including pain, bleeding, compression of vital organ systems, ulcerating skin lesions, skeletal and brain metastases

(2) While external beam radiation is the modality commonly used for palliative radiation therapy, an intravenous radioactive medication such as strontium-89, phosphorus 32, or samarium 153 may also be used for bone disease

f) Oncologic emergencies—radiation therapy is the treatment of choice for spinal cord compression, and frequently in superior vena cava syndrome and symptomatic brain metastases

3. Chemotherapy

a) Definition: the systemic treatment of disease by medication

(1) Initially used in the treatment of infectious disease, and currently is most commonly used in the context of cancer treatment

(2) The use of chemotherapy for cancer treatment is based on cellular kinetics, which include cell life cycle, cell cycle time, growth fraction and overall tumor burden

(3) There are over 50 chemotherapeutic agents in current use with more in the development phases

(4) Often used in combination to achieve better response by affecting various phases of cellular growth and to reduce toxic effects

b) Chemotherapy is used to treat cancer in three ways:

(1) Cure—either by chemotherapy alone or in combination with other cancer treatment modalities, such as surgery, radiation

(2) Control—to extend the length and quality of life when cure is not a realistic goal

(3) Palliation—to improve or enhance comfort when neither cure nor control are possible. Examples include relief of pressure on nerves, lymphatics, and blood vessels and reduction in organ obstruction

c) Side effects of chemotherapy; vary from one drug to another and most can be prevented[3]

(1) Short-term side effects, generally lasting a few days

(a) Nausea and vomiting—from denuded GI epithelium and stimulation of Chemoreceptor Trigger Zone (CTZ) in the emetic center of the brain

(b) Diarrhea—resulting from denuded epithelium in the bowel and subsequent inflammation

(c) Anorexia and stomatitis—from denuded epithelium and subsequent inflammation; anorexia may have already existed from the cancer itself

    (d) Bone marrow suppression

        (i) Neutropenia—making the patient susceptible to infection

        (ii) Thrombocytopenia—making the patient susceptible to bleeding problems

        (iii) Anemia usually results after several cycles of chemotherapy because of the long life-span of red blood cells (120 days). These same patients also frequently develop anemia of chronic disease.

  (2) Long-term side effects

    (a) Neurotoxicity—from drugs such as plant alkaloids, etoposide, taxanes, platinum compounds

        (i) Peripheral nerve damage can result in varying degrees of numbness in toes and legs first, which may lead to stumbling causing inadvertent injury, then in fingers

        (ii) Constipation can result when nerve endings in the bowel are affected

    (b) Nephrotoxicity (acute tubular necrosis)—from drugs such as cisplatin, high dose methotrexate or streptozocin

        (i) Usually prevented by adequate hydration

        (ii) Once tubular necrosis occurs, some degree of renal failure will persist

    (c) Cardiotoxicity resulting in irreversible cardiomyopathy—from drugs such as doxorubicin and daunomycin

    (d) Hemorrhagic cystitis—usually from cyclophosphamide

        (i) Usually prevented by adequate fluid intake and frequent bladder emptying

        (ii) Once it occurs, patient will have chronic flair-ups of cystitis (dysuria, frequency, urgency and/or hematuria)

    (e) Pulmonary fibrosis—long term effects of bleomycin

E. Supportive treatments

1. Blood component therapy, antimicrobial therapy, nutritional support (parenteral or enteral), hydration and supplementation for metabolic and chemistry abnormalities

2. Complementary Therapies—psychological techniques, supplements and herbs, support groups

3. Unproven Therapies—unproven in animal or human trials, usually expensive to the patient because they are not covered by insurance

F.   The major cancer diagnoses*

   1.   Lung cancer (16% of new cancer diagnoses; Lung cancer is the leading cause of cancer death—31% of all cancer deaths)

     a)   Indications of advanced disease: cough, hemoptysis, dyspnea, pneumonia, shoulder pain, arm pain, superior vena cava syndrome, Syndrome of Inappropriate Antidiuretic Hormone (SIADH)

     b)   Unique issues: cures are very rare (13% long term survival greater than 5 years), often advanced at diagnosis; association with smoking and tobacco use, small cell variety may present with brain metastasis

     c)   Social/psychological issues: social isolation, limited survival, rapid family role changes and disruptions, guilt over smoking

   2.   Breast cancer (31% of new cancer diagnoses; 15% of cancer deaths)

     a)   Indications of advanced disease:

       (1)   Local—painless mass, dimpling of skin, nipple retraction or deviation, asymmetry of breasts, scaling of skin on nipple or areola, peau d'orange skin (skin takes on a porous thickening, similar to the skin of an orange), bloody or serous discharge from nipple, ulceration of the breast

       (2)   Metastatic—bone, brain, liver

     b)   Unique issues—sexuality, femininity; body image changes, genetic susceptibility

   3.   Genitourinary cancers

     a)   Prostate cancer (15% of new cancer diagnoses; 7% of cancer deaths)

       (1)   Indications of advanced disease:

         (a)   Local: hematuria, painful defecation, obstructive urinary symptoms, weight loss

         (b)   Metastatic: appear generally debilitated, older than chronological age and may present with bone and neuropathic pain from bone involvement or nerve compression, weight loss, lethargy, and secondary disease (pneumonia, etc.)

     b)   Bladder cancer (4% of new cancer diagnoses; 2% of cancer deaths)

       (1)   Indications of advanced disease: hematuria, decrease in force or caliber of urine stream, flank pain, hydronephrosis, renal failure

       (2)   Unique issues: surgical resection in males may cause impotence, in females the anterior wall of the vagina may be removed; body image changes if stomas are present, sexuality

     c)   Kidney cancer (2% of new cancer diagnoses; 2% of cancer deaths)

       (1)   Indications of advanced disease: gross hematuria, pain (dull aching), palpable abdominal mass, fever, weight loss, elevated erythrocyte sedimentation rate (ESR), and/or anemia, dyspnea

---

* Estimates of new cases and deaths for the cancer diagnoses listed below are from the American Cancer Society's publication, *Cancer Facts and Figures—2001.*

(2)   Unique issues: approx. 30–50% of patients have metastatic disease at diagnosis; associated with cigarette smoking and occupational exposure to asbestos, cadmium, and lead

(3)   Unique issues: some patients exhibit signs and symptoms of bone marrow involvement, anemia, blood loss, and tendency to hemorrhage, sexual dysfunction, surgical or medical castration may cause psychological sequelae

4.   Reproductive cancers

a)   Ovarian cancer (2% of new cancer diagnoses; 2.5% of cancer deaths)

(1)   Indications of advanced disease: palpable abdominal or pelvic mass, ascites, increased abdominal girth, pleural effusions, intestinal obstruction, weight loss

(2)   Unique issues: majority of cases are diagnosed at later stages

b)   Endometrial cancer (3% of new cancer diagnoses; 1% of cancer deaths)

(1)   Indications of advanced disease: hemorrhage, ascites, jaundice, bowel obstruction, dyspnea

(2)   Unique issues: sexual dysfunction; disease difficult to treat with distant metastasis

c)   Cervical cancer (1% of new cancer diagnoses; less than 1% of cancer deaths)

(1)   Indications of advanced disease: dyspareunia, urinary symptoms (dysuria, urinary retention, urinary frequency, hematuria), bowel symptoms (rectal bleeding, constipation, bowel obstruction), abdominal or pelvic pain referred to flank or leg, lower extremity edema

(2)   Unique issues: advanced disease upon diagnosis, sexuality; body image, guilt if not doing regular PAP smears

d)   Testicular cancer (less than 1% of new cancer diagnoses; less than 1% of cancer deaths)

(1)   Indications of advanced disease: back pain, bone pain, dyspnea, seizures, headache, cough

(2)   Unique issues: early signs and symptoms are usually absent; because testicular cancer is often curable even in later stages, patients and families may have issues associated with treatment failure

5.   Gastrointestinal cancers

a)   Colon, rectal and anal cancers (11% of new cancer diagnoses; 10% of cancer deaths)

(1)   Indications of advanced disease: constipation, incontinence, weight loss, sensation of rectal fullness, dull or aching perineal or sacral pain often radiating down the legs; cutaneous manifestations, rectal-vaginal fistula, rectal bleeding

(2)   Symptoms of metastatic disease: pulmonary (cough, chest pain, dyspnea, hemoptysis, wheezing, dysphagia), hepatic (ascites, abdominal distention, nausea, anorexia, increasing abdominal girth, changes in color of urine and stool, pruritis)

(3)   Unique issues: common cancer site; may be perceived as preventable; body image secondary to colostomy or ileul conduits

b)   Esophagus (1% of new cancer diagnoses; 2% of cancer deaths)

(1)   Indications of advanced disease: progressive dysphagia or airway obstruction (often with need for gastrostomy or jejunostomy), dehydration, general debilitation, larger tumors can cause aspiration

(2)   Unique issues: grows and disseminates rapidly, advanced disease upon diagnosis, nutritional issues,

c)   Liver (1% of new cancer diagnoses; 2% of cancer deaths)

(1)   Indications of advanced disease: hepatic failure, severe ascites, infection, predisposition to bleeding, pain, weight loss, weakness, pneumonia, anorexia, nausea, vomiting, muscle atrophy, confusion, dyspnea, pruritis, jaundice, peripheral edema, immobility with its sequelae

(2)   Unique issues: frequently associated with cirrhosis, aggressive disease course

d)   Stomach (2% of new cancer diagnoses; 2% of cancer deaths)

(1)   Indications of advanced disease: enzyme and nutritional deficiencies, malnutrition, weakness, immobility

(2)   Unique issues: most patients die of bronchopneumonia or lung abscess secondary to immobility and malnutrition; deep vein thrombosis and pulmonary embolism secondary to immobility are also common causes of death; nutritional concerns

e)   Pancreas (2% of new cancer diagnoses; 5% of cancer deaths)

(1)   Indications of advanced disease: hepatic failure, ascites, severe jaundice, hemorrhage, infection, abdominal pain, especially neuropathic pain related to invasion of the celiac plexus, anorexia, nausea, vomiting, diarrhea, early satiety

(2)   Unique issues: early symptoms are vague and mimic common gastrointestinal illnesses, advanced disease upon diagnosis

6.   Leukemias/hematological malignancies

a)   Leukemia (2% of new cancer diagnoses; 4% of cancer deaths)

(1)   Indications of advanced disease: bruising, bleeding from nose, gums, bladder or bowel, fatigue, recurrent or persistent infection, fevers, disseminated intravascular coagulation

(2)   Unique issues: emotional ups and down related to multiple remission inductions and relapses, necessity for long periods of treatment, possible failure of bone marrow transplantation

b)   Multiple Myeloma (1% of new cancer diagnoses; 2% of cancer deaths)

(1)   Indications of advanced disease: infections, pain, hypercalcemia, pathologic fractures, decreased mobility, anemia, decreased platelets, bleeding tendencies, renal insufficiency, hyperuricemia, constipation

(2)   Unique issues: leading cause of death is bone marrow failures, infections, respiratory and renal failure; patients may experience long periods of latent disease

      c)   Lymphomas (5% of new cancer diagnoses; 5% of cancer deaths)

           (1)   Indications of advanced disease: fever, night sweats, weight loss, decrease in urinary output, itching, lower back pain, shortness of breath, pruritis, adenopathy

           (2)   Unique issues: some types are highly treatable and curable

7.   Melanoma (3% of new cancer diagnoses; 1% of cancer deaths; incidence has doubled in last 20 years)

      a)   Indications of advanced disease: depend on site of distant metastasis (most common sites are liver, lung, bone, and brain)

      b)   Unique issues: metastatic disease is highly resistant to systemic chemotherapy; patient and family may have issues regarding prevention, diagnosis

8.   Head and Neck cancers (4% of new cancer diagnoses; 3% of cancer deaths)

      a)   Indications of advanced disease: local extension, formation of fistulas, wound breakdown, potential for carotid artery rupture (occurs in approx. 3.5% of patients with head and neck cancer, pain (described often as throbbing, pounding, pressure-like), dysphagia, increase in neck lymph nodes, ulceration, airway obstruction, bone pain

      b)   Unique issues: disfigurement, self image, depression, social isolation, many patients have reconstructive surgery; presence of tracheostomy, inability to speak

9.   Brain tumors (1% of new cancer diagnoses; 2% of cancer deaths)

      a)   Indications of advanced disease: increased intracranial pressure

           (1)   *Beginning late-stage signs:* drowsiness, decreased attention span, mood changes, poor judgment, impaired cognitive skills, short term memory

           (2)   *End-stage signs and symptoms:* headache, vomiting, papilledema, decreased level of consciousness, changes in vital signs, including widening of pulse pressure, bradycardia, slowed, irregular pulse, displacement of brain structures (herniation), seizures, personality changes, loss of sensation, disturbances in coordination, malnutrition and dehydration

      b)   Unique issues: prognosis has not changed in last 10 years; many symptoms drastically affect normal functioning

G.   Oncologic Emergencies and Complications

1.   For any of these life-threatening complications, interventions should be determined only after:

      a)   Considering where the patient is along the disease trajectory

      b)   Clarifying goals of treatment with patient and family

      c)   Helping patient and family to arrive at attainable goals

      d)   Considering how likely is it that the treatment will result in hoped-for outcomes

2.   Central Nervous System

    a)   Spinal Cord Compression

        (1)   Pressure on cord resulting in loss of nerve function or vertebral collapse

        (2)   Caused by neoplastic invasion or cord ischemia secondary to collapse of vertebra

        (3)   Signs and Symptoms

            (a)   Localized back pain may be only symptom prior to complete paralysis

            (b)   Motor deficits—hypotonicity, hyperflexia, paralysis

            (c)   Sensory deficits—paresthesia, bowel and bladder incontinence

        (4)   Requires emergent treatment (unless contra-indicated by patient condition or preferences)

            (a)   High dose corticosteriods

            (b)   MRI

            (c)   Radiation

            (d)   Surgical consult for decompression and stabilization

    b)   Intracerebral Metastases

        (1)   Causes increased intracranial pressure

        (2)   Signs and Symptoms

            (a)   Early morning headache

            (b)   Cognitive dysfunction

            (c)   Confusion

            (d)   Projectile vomiting

        (3)   Treatment

            (a)   Corticosteriods

            (b)   Whole brain radiation

            (c)   Sometimes surgical removal of single lesion

3.   Metabolic/Endocrine

    a)   SIADH (Syndrome of Inappropriate Antidiuretic Hormone)

        (1)   Caused by excessive antidiuretic hormone from the posterior pituitary gland. Can be medication induced

        (2)   Signs and symptoms include hyponatremia, weight gain, nausea, vomiting, CNS changes, weakness, lethargy, irritability, confusion, diarrhea, muscle cramps, convulsions

        (3)   Treatment (if patient can tolerate and desirable effects can be obtained)

            (a)   Fluid restriction

            (b)   Hypertonic saline

            (c)   Furosemide (Lasix®)

            (d)   Demeclocycline (Declomycin®)

b)   Hypercalcemia

        (1)   Caused by increased calcium levels from cancer involvement of the bone; serum calcium greater than 11 (may be lower if albumin is low as calcium is bound to protein)

        (2)   Signs and symptoms include nausea, vomiting, anorexia, constipation, lethargy, confusion polyuria, stupor, coma, mental status changes, polydipsia

        (3)   Treatment may include

            (a)   Hydration

            (b)   Furosemide (Lasix®)

            (c)   Bone resorption inhibitors (bisphosphonates such as pamidronate, (Aredia®), etridronate (Didronel®), etc.)

            (d)   Steroids

c)   Tumor Lysis Syndrome

        (1)   Caused by rapid release of intracellular potassium, phosphate and nucleic acid into the blood stream, resulting in electrolyte imbalance

        (2)   Signs and symptoms are hyperkalemia, hyperphosphatemia, hyperuricemia, hypocalcemia, neuromuscular changes, twitching, renal failure

        (3)   Treatment/prevention (if patient can tolerate and desirable effects can be obtained)

            (a)   Hydration

            (b)   Diuretics

            (c)   Allopurinol (Zyloprim®)

d)   Septic Shock

        (1)   Caused by cardiovascular collapse in response to toxins in the blood

        (2)   Signs and symptoms include fever, chills, warm skin progressing to cold, clammy skin, hypotension, mental status changes, oliguria

        (3)   Treatment (if patient can tolerate and desirable effects can be obtained)

            (a)   Fluid replacement

            (b)   Antibiotics

            (c)   Vasoconstrictive medications

            (d)   Oxygen

e)   Anaphylaxis

(1)   Caused by immediate sensitivity reaction caused by chemotherapy, biological response modifiers and some medications

(2)   Signs and symptoms include respiratory distress, hypertension, fainting, itching bradycardia, tachycardia and respiratory arrest

(3)   Treatment is emergent

(a)   Epinephrine (Adrenaline®)

(b)   Diphenhydramine (Benadryl®)

(c)   Hydrocortisone (Cortef®)

(d)   Airway maintenance

(e)   CPR, if appropriate

4.   Cardiovascular/Hematologic

a)   Carotid Artery Rupture—most often a terminal event

(1)   Caused by tumor invasion or erosion of arterial wall due to neoplastic tumor, radiation necrosis, infection or poor wound healing

(2)   Signs and symptoms include tumor involvement around the artery, pulsating tumor, exposure of artery, minor oozing to major hemorrhage, anxiety, decreased blood pressure, respiratory distress

(3)   Treatment focuses on supporting patient and family

(a)   Patient/family education to potential terminal event—dark towels should be available to apply to sight if needed

(b)   Prefilled syringes of pain medications and benzodiazepines available to sedate patient if time allows

(c)   Sandbag to apply pressure to site

(d)   Treat areas of oozing with topical epinephrine

(e)   Use dark colored towels to manage bleeding

b)   Cardiac Tamponade

(1)   Caused by excessive accumulation of blood or fluid around pericardium, which prevents adequate pumping of ventricles

(2)   Signs and symptoms include retrosternal chest pain, dysphagia, cough, dyspnea, hoarseness, increased jugular venous pressure, muffled heart sounds, pericardial friction rub, tachycardia, and pulsus paradoxus

(3)   Requires emergent treatment (unless contra indicated by patient condition or preferences)

(a)   Pericardiocentesis

(b)   High dose steroids

(c)   Diuretics

        (d)   Oxygen

        (e)   Radiation

c)   SVCS (Superior Vena Cava Syndrome)

    (1)   Caused by venous congestion secondary to obstruction in upper thorax, common in lung and breast cancer, lymphomas, brain tumors, and tumors compressing on chest wall

    (2)   Signs and symptoms include dyspnea, headache, visual disturbances, facial edema, jugular distention, swelling of trunk and upper extremities, chest pain, and cough

    (3)   Treatment (depending on disease trajectory and patient goals)

        (a)   Steroids

        (b)   Diuretics

        (c)   Thrombolytic therapy

        (d)   Radiation

        (e)   Chemotherapy

d)   DIC (Disseminated Intravascular Coagulation)

    (1)   Caused by the process of generalized activation of hemostatis, which results in widespread fibrin formation, followed by lysis within the vascular system

    (2)   Signs and symptoms include bleeding and clotting, ecchymosis, petechiae and purpura, dyspnea, restlessness, altered LOC, tachycardia

    (3)   Treatment is controversial since clotting and bleeding must be treated simultaneously; best managed by treating underlying malignancy. Can also present as a low level, chronic disease

        (a)   Blood component therapy

        (b)   Antiembolic medications including heparin, Antithrombin II, and fibrinolytic inhibitors

        (c)   Hydration

        (d)   Oxygen

        (e)   Anxiolytics

5.   Gastrointestinal: Bowel Obstruction

a)   Caused by tumor blocking bowel causing normal transit in the intestinal tract to be delayed or prevented

b)   Signs and Symptoms include pain, nausea, vomiting, constipation, diarrhea, abdominal distention

c)   Treatment

    (1)   Surgery if appropriate

    (2)   Nasogastric suction or venting gastrostomy

    (3)   IV fluids, if appropriate

(4)   Pain Medications

(5)   Steroids

(6)   Octreotide (Sandostatin®) 100–600 mcg/day by subcutaneous injection

III. Neurological Conditions

A. Pathophysiology

1. Injury:

   a) Cerebrovascular Accident (CVA) Leading cause of serious long-term disability and third leading cause of death in U.S.

   b) Cerebral cell death occurs in localized areas due to embolic materials clogging a vessel, vessel rupture from aneurysm or hypertension, infections, or plaques in cerebral blood vessels that diminish blood flow

   c) Damage depends on size and location; sequelae range from none to irreversible comatose state and/or brain death

2. Trauma:

   a) Injury to skull, with intracranial or subdural bleeding, and prolonged high ICP (intracranial pressure), leads to damage in patterns similar to CVAs

   b) Central Nervous System Anoxia: Global CNS anoxia following cardiopulmonary arrest can result in a persistent vegetative state

3. Degenerative Diseases

   a) Motor Neuron Disease: Amyotrophic Lateral Sclerosis (ALS)*: A degenerative disease of the motor neurons in the cerebral cortex, brainstem and spinal cord, resulting in progressive weakness and atrophy of striated muscles. Usually there is no change in intellectual function

   b) Dementia: Dementia of the Alzheimer's Type (DAT): An irreversible and progressive dementia characterized by intellectual deterioration, disorganization of the personality, and inability to carry out the tasks of daily living. Multi-infarct dementia can mimic some aspects of Alzheimer's Disease

B. Primary Treatment of Disease

1. Pharmacologic:

   a) CVA: TPA within 3 hours of stroke, anticoagulants during the acute phase; diuretics to reduce cerebral edema, anticonvulsants for seizure control; antihypertensives and ASA for subsequent CVA prevention

   b) Trauma: Management of increased ICP with corticosteroids and mannitol in acute phases

   c) CNS anoxia: No treatment available

---

* With thanks to Kathy Roelke, RN, Nurse Clinician-3, Neurology and ALS Clinic, University of Wisconsin Hospitals and Clinics, Madison, WI

Patterns of Metastatic Spread⁴—Common Sites of Metastases

Primary Disease	bone	marrow	skin	Lung	Liver	bowel rectum	NODES	kidney GU	Brain meninges	peritoneal	adrenal glands
bladder							X	X	X	X	
brain									X		
breast	X*	X		X*	X*		X*		X*		
cervix	X			X	X	X	X	X			
colon				X*	X*		X*	X			
esophagus	X			X	X		X*				X
head/neck			X	X*			X				
hepatoma	X			X			X				
kidney	X		X	X	X		X		X		
Leukemia/lymphoma	X	X	X	X			X		X		
lung	X*	X*			X*		X*	X	X*		
melanoma	X*	X	X	X*	X*		X*		X		
ovary				X*	X*	X	X*			X*	
pancreas				X	X	X	X				
prostate	X	X		X	X		X				
sarcoma				X*	X*		X*				
stomach	X			X	X		X				
testes	X			X	X		X				
thyroid	X			X			X				
uterus	X									X	

*Most common sites of metastasis • Cancers that spread to **brain**: breast, cervix, esophagus, liver, kidney, lung, melanoma, prostate, stomach, testes, thyroid • All spread to **lung** *except*: bladder, brain and uterus • Cancers that spread to **bone**: breast, kidney, lung, melanoma

        d)   ALS: none have been identified effective; experimental trials are ongoing

        e)   Alzheimer's: experimental drugs include cholinergic, dopamine and serotonin precursors; neuropeptides; and transcerebral dilators; haloperidol and anxiolytics help control agitation

        f)   Functional:

            (1)   Re-establish or maintain simple and routine ADLs

            (2)   Build on, or adapt ADLs as possible and necessary

            (3)   Nutritional support

            (4)   Prevention of complications related to immobility

        g)   Psychological/social

C.   Indications of Advanced Disease

1.   Injury: CVA, Trauma and CNS anoxia result in permanent neurological deficits that predispose the patient to complications, particularly impaired mobility, dysphagia and incontinence; death usually results from untreated or refractory infection, or from general malnutrition even with the use of feeding tubes; in the case of post-CVA patients, subsequent CVAs may cause death

2.   Degenerative Diseases:

        a)   ALS: Progressive muscle weakness eventually affects all striated muscles except sphincters and extraocular muscles

            (1)   Common symptoms include cramps, atrophy of one or more extremities, fasciculations, hyper-reflexia, dysphagia, dyspnea and impaired speech

            (2)   Although choking spells are common and distressing in the last stages of ALS, it is rarely the cause of death

            (3)   Involvement of respiratory muscles and subsequent upper respiratory infections generally leads to sudden deterioration and death

            (4)   Treat with aggressive psychological support

        b)   Alzheimer's Disease: With disease progression, performance of ADLs becomes impossible, and the patient eventually becomes bed bound

            (1)   Problems in late disease include incontinence, loss of speech, myocolonic jerking, seizure activity and loss of consciousness

            (2)   Death is usually a result of complications related to immobility

IV. Cardiac Conditions

A. Pathophysiology

1.   Cardiovascular disease is the single leading cause of death in America today

2.   Cardiomyopathies: A diverse group of primary myocardial diseases

        a)   About half of the cases are idiopathic

b) Others can be attributed to chronic, high alcohol intake, auto-immune processes, viral infections, inherited tendencies, inflammatory processes, metabolic and endocrine diseases, exposure to toxins and selected medications (including some chemotherapeutic agents), infiltrative diseases (amyloidosis, sarcoidosis), fibroplastic diseases, hypersensitivity to selected medications, and coronary artery disease

c) Presents as either diffuse degeneration of myocardial fibers, hypertrophy of the myocardium, or infiltration of the myocardium with fibrous tissue, resulting in decreased cardiac output

3. Coronary Artery Disease (CAD): Also referred to as heart disease

a) A state in which one or more of the coronary arteries has a narrowing of the lumen resulting in loss of oxygen to the myocardium and causing the symptoms of ischemia, angina, or myocardial infarction

b) Underlying pathology of CAD is accumulation of atherosclerotic lesions which adhere to the smooth muscle of the coronary artery and are made up of connective tissue and intracellular and extracellular lipids

B. Treatment

1. Surgical

a) For cardiomyopathies, only surgical treatment is heart transplant. Hospice and palliative care programs will occasionally care for persons with rejected or failed heart transplants

b) For CAD, angioplasty or bypass surgery attempt to permanently increase coronary blood flow. In some cases agents are tried

2. Pharmacologic:

a) For cardiomyopathy, drug therapies include cardiac glycosides to increase cardiac contractility (digitalis); Pre-load reducers (diuretics, nitrates, morphine); After-load reducers (ACE inhibitors and calcium channel blockers)

b) For CAD, drug therapies are nitrates for vasodilation and improved blood flow; calcium channel blockers to reduce cardiac afterload; ACE inhibitors which also reduce left cardiac afterload; Beta blockers to decrease heart rate and oxygen demand

3. Other treatment modalities:

a) Cardiac rehab programs/safe exercise

b) Diet/weight loss, e.g., heart-healthy and/or low sodium diet

c) Optimal reduction of all risk factors

d) Stress management programs

e) Lifestyle adaptation

C. **Indications of Advanced Disease**

1. Congestive heart failure (CHF) is defined as the inability of the heart to supply the heart muscle itself and the rest of the body with adequate arterial pressure and circulatory volume. Initially, it may occur on the right or left side of the heart, but eventually both sides are affected

2. CHF also activates the cyclo-angiotension-aldersterone system causing salt and water retention, arteriolar vasoconstriction, and increased cardiac afterload. Sodium retention is a chief feature in the pathology of CHF

3. Left-sided congestive heart failure initially causes congestion in the lungs and has the following signs and symptoms:

   a) Anxiety and restlessness

   b) Dyspnea

   c) Orthopnea, paroxysmal nocturnal dyspnea

   d) Cough, hemoptysis

   e) Tachycardia, palpitations

   f) Basilar rales, bronchial wheezes

   g) Fatigue, decreased exercise tolerance

   h) Cyanosis (a late sign of hypoxia in adults) or pallor

4. Right-sided congestive heart failure causes congestion in the systemic circulation, most notable in the lower extremities and liver and has the following signs and symptoms:

   a) Anorexia, nausea

   b) Weight gain

   c) Nocturia, oliguria

   d) Dependent peripheral edema

   e) Weakness

D. **Unique issues**

1. Perception that with heart disease there is always something more that can be done

2. Symptom management can and likely will prolong the patient's life

3. The "ups and downs" of the disease (exacerbations) keep patient and family thinking that the patient will "recover" again

V. **Pulmonary Conditions**

A. **Pathophysiology**

1. Obstructive pulmonary diseases: Chronic spasm of small airways due to chronic disease, toxin, and tobacco exposure; forced expiratory volume (FEV1) is reduced and chest is chronically hyperinflated; Pco_2 increased; Po_2 drops

2. There are two types of obstructive lung disease, each with its own unique presentation

    a) Type A COPD (Emphysema)

        (1) Patient is typically thin; muscle wasting

        (2) Absence of central cyanosis

        (3) Use of accessory muscles for breathing

        (4) "Barrel chest" appearance

        (5) Decreased ability to cough effectively

        (6) Hyper-resonance on percussion

        (7) Distant, diminished breath sounds

    b) Type B COPD (Chronic bronchitis)

        (1) Patient is typically overweight

        (2) Central cyanosis is present

        (3) Minimal use of accessory muscles

        (4) Resonance on percussion

        (5) Adventitious breath sounds, typically wheezes

3. Restrictive pulmonary diseases

    a) Defined as loss of lung tissue or limited lung expansion due to decreased compliance of the lung or muscle weakness; forced vital capacity (FVC) and vital capacity are less than 80% of normal predicted value

    b) Examples: pectus excavatum, myasthenia gravis, diffuse idiopathic interstitial fibrosis, and space occupying lesions (effusions, tumors)

B. Treatment Modalities:

1. Pharmacologic:

    a) For obstructive lung disease: xanthines and other bronchodilators, corticosteroids, anticholinergics by IV, oral, topical routes; nebulizer treatments; oxygen is less helpful, but can provide comfort; antibiotic therapy may be used to treat infections if appropriate

    b) For restrictive lung disease: corticosteroids, oxygen; respiratory therapies/Nebulizers/IPPB; antibiotic therapy may be used to treat infections if appropriate

C. Indications of Advanced Disease

1. Cor Pulmonale:

    a) Both types of lung failure cause an increase in pulmonary pressure, which can lead first to right ventricular failure (cor pulmonale), then to left ventricular failure

    b) Can present as acute or chronic

2.   Respiratory Failure:

a)   Both types of lung disease eventually result in lungs that are unable to meet the needs of life

b)   Low P_{O_2} and high P_{CO_2} leads to chronic fatigue, very limited tolerance to physical exertion, profound feeling of breathlessness, and poor quality of life

VI. Renal Conditions

A.   Pathophysiology

1.   Renal Failure: the causes of acute and chronic renal failure are the same; the onset of chronic is slower and more insidious

a)   Can be oliguric or non-oliguric

b)   BUN and creatinine rise

2.   Causes include: toxins; nephrotoxic medications (e.g., cis-platinum, gentamicin); infiltrative malignant processes (e.g., cyclov, metastatic tumor); metabolic ion overload (e.g., hypercalcemia or uricemia); infectious processes (e.g., glomerulonephritis); collagen vascular disease (e.g., lupus, scleroderma); diabetes, hypertension

B.   Treatment modalities

1.   Dialysis: Peritoneal or Hemodialysis

a)   Useful short term in acute renal failure

b)   Provides renal cells a chance to regenerate

c)   May also be required long term with permanent kidney damage

2.   Surgical Intervention

a)   Many surgical procedures available to relieve obstruction, ranging from simple nephrostomy tubes to major tumor debulking with ostomies

b)   Procedures chosen, if any, depend on goals of the patient and family, goals of treatment based on the disease trajectory, and quality of life

3.   Pharmacologic Interventions: For chronic renal failure, diuretics are often prescribed; high phosphate levels are often treated with aluminum gels such as Aluminum Hydroxide, as well as phosphate binders such as Calcium Acetate

4.   Nutritional Interventions: Low sodium, low protein, low potassium and/or low phosphate diet, if applicable based on the course of the disease trajectory

C.   Indications of Advanced Disease

1.   Fluid and Electrolyte Imbalances

a)   With increasing renal insufficiency, patients may become oliguric requiring fluid restriction with increased doses of diuretics; most patients require sodium restriction

b)   Potassium restriction is usually necessary; hyperkalemia is frequent and can be life threatening; patients who choose to allow K^+ to rise to lethal levels usually experience profound muscle weakness and death from arrhythmia

c)   Anemias: with associated dyspnea, chest pain, weakness

d)   Uremia: symptoms of end-stage uremia include renal osteodystrophy (bone pain, fractures, skeletal deformity, proximal muscle), severe pruritis, CHF and coronary insufficiency; hypertension; uremic encephalopathy develops as condition worsens and as death approaches

VII. Gastrointestinal Conditions

A. Pathophysiology

1.   See also Gastrointestinal Cancers in Section II of this chapter

2.   Hepatic failure: A number of liver diseases can lead to hepatocellular injury and cirrhosis, including alcoholic liver disease, chronic hepatitis, viral infections, autoimmune diseases, drug toxicities, metabolic causes

B. Treatment

1.   Treat underlying disease to extent possible

2.   Transplant

3.   Manage symptoms for comfort only

C. Indications of Advanced Disease

1.   Esophageal varices (along with portal hypertension and abnormal coagulation); this is a major risk for hemorrhage

2.   Ascites (major risk is spontaneous bacterial peritonitis and respiratory compromise)

3.   Hepatic encephalopathy

4.   Other symptoms may include jaundice, pruritis, anorexia, nausea and liver capsule pain

VIII. General Debility

A. Pathophysiology

1.   Debility, unspecified, is a diagnostic category for elderly, debilitated patients with functional disabilities and progressive multiple organ failure who do not meet criteria for a specific terminal illness.

a)   In the past, the pediatric diagnosis "failure to thrive" has been used for this condition

b)   There is now an ICD-9 Code (783.7) for use with adult patients[5]

2.   Severe functional deficits in activities of daily living (ADLs)

3.   Low Karnofsky performance scores

4. Signs and symptoms of multiple organ impairment and impending failure

5. Progressive physical deterioration

B. Treatment

1. Symptom management

2. Appropriate nutritional support

3. Prevention of complications related to immobility

C. Indications of Advanced Disease: Terminal phase consistent with organ failure and complications of immobility

IX. Endocrine Disorders

A. Pathophysiology

1. Diabetes Mellitus (DM): Leading cause of chronic renal failure

2. Persistent hyperglycemia related to an inability to produce or utilize insulin to meet metabolic demand

    a) Insulin Dependent (Type I) DM

        (1) Usual onset in children and young adults, but can occur at any age

        (2) Research suggests an autoimmune process that progressively destroys pancreatic beta cells causes Type I DM; the body is unable to produce insulin, and exogenous insulin is necessary for survival

    b) Non-insulin dependent (Type II) DM

        (1) Usual onset after age 30

        (2) Type II DM is caused by impairment in the pancreatic insulin release sites or a diminished number of peripheral receptor sites, leading to insulin resistance; exogenous insulin is not necessary to sustain life, but may be given to treat hyperglycemia

    c) Other (secondary) DM: Hyperglycemia related to another cause, such as pancreatic disease or medication effects

B. Treatment: Directed to maintaining glycemic control through insulin or oral anti-diabetic drugs, dietary modifications, blood glucose monitoring and patient teaching

C. Indications of Advanced Disease

1. Diabetic ketoacidosis in Type I DM or nonketotic hyperglycemic-hyperosmolar coma in Type II DM can result in death at any time in the disease process

2. Chronic, life-limiting complications can occur in all types of DM, and there is strong evidence that poor glycemic control is directly related to their development

3. Complications include:

    a) Diabetic retinopathy

    b) Peripheral vascular and coronary artery disease

    c) Diabetic enteropathy with impaired GI motility

    d) Diabetic neuropathy

    e) Autonomic neuropathy, which can cause postural hypotension, persistent tachycardia, neurogenic bladder, incontinence of urine or feces, diabetic nephropathy, resulting in hypertension and ultimately, renal failure

    f) Recurrent infections and impaired wound healing

REFERENCES

1. Sherman, D.W., *Patients with acquired immune deficiency syndrome,* in *Oxford textbook of palliative nursing,* B.R. Ferrell and N. Coyle, Editors. 2001, Oxford University Press: New York.

2. American Cancer Society, *Cancer facts and figures 2002.* 2002, American Center Society.

3. Yarbro, C.H., et al., *Cancer nursing: Principles and practice.* 5th Edition ed, ed. C.H. Yarbro, et al. 2000, Sudbury, MA: Jones and Bartlett.

4. Volker, B., *Hospice and Palliative Nurses Practice Review.* 3rd Edition ed, ed. B. Volker. 1999, Dubuque, IA: Kendall/Hunt Publishing.

5. American Medical Association, *International classification of disease.* 9th ed. 2001, Chicago: AMA Press.

GENERAL REFERENCES

Ahya, S.N., Flood, L., and Paranjothi, S., (Eds.) (2001). *The Washington manual of medical therapeutics.* St. Louis: Washington University School of Medicine.

Berger, AM, Portenoy, RK, Weissman, DE. (Eds.) (1998). *Principles and practice of supportive oncology.* Philadelphia: Lippincott, Williams, and Wilkins.

Borasio, G.D., and Voltz, R. (1997, October). Palliative care in amyotrophic lateral sclerosis. *Journal of Neurology.* (Suppl. 4), S11–17.

Borasio, G.D., and Voltz, R. (1997 October). Palliative therapy in the terminal stage of neurological disease. *Journal of Neurology.* (Suppl. 4), S2–10.

Boswell, S.L. (1995). Outpatient management of HIV infection in the adult: An update, *Current Clinical Topics in Infectious Diseases, 15*:30–43.

Ciezki, JP, Komurcu, S, and Macklis, R. (2000). Palliative radiotherapy. *Seminars in Oncology.* Vol 27(1): 90–93.

Dow, KH, Bucholtz, JD, Iwamoto, R, Fieler, V, and Hilderly, L (1997). *Nursing care in radiation oncology,* (2nd. Ed.). W. B. Saunders, Co. Philadelphia.

Doyle, D., Hanks, G.W.C., and MacDonald, N., eds. (1998). *Oxford textbook of palliative medicine.* (2nd ed.). New York: Oxford University Press.

Dunne-Daly, C. (1999) Principles of radiotherapy and radiobiology. *Seminars in Oncology Nursing Vol 15*(4):250–259.

Haylock, PJ (1998). Cancer metastasis: An update. *Seminars in Oncology Nursing.* 14(3):172–177.

Kirton, CA, Ferri, RS, and Eleftherakis, V. (1999). Primary care and case management of the patient with AIDS. *Nursing Clinics of North America.* 34(1):71–93.

Langford, R., and Thompson, J. Eds. (2000). *Mosby's handbook of diseases.* St. Louis: Mosby.

National Hospice Organization. (1996). *Medical guidelines for determining prognosis in selected non-cancer diseases.* (2nd ed.). Arlington, VA: Author.

Nelson, KA, Walsh D, Abdullan O, McDonnell F, Homsi J, Komucurcu, S., LeGrand, Zhuovsky, D. (2000). Common complications of advanced cancer. *Seminars in Oncology,* 27(1):34–44.

Newshan, G. and Sherman, DW. (1999). Palliative care—pain symptom management in persons with HIV/AIDS. *Nursing Clinics of North America.* 34(1): 131–145.

Oliver, D., Borasio, G.D., and Walsh, D. (eds.). (2000). *Palliative care in amyotrophic lateral sclerosis.* Oxford: Oxford University Press.

O'Mahony, S, Coyle, N., and Payne, R. (2000). Multidisciplinary care of the terminally ill patient. *Surgical Clinics of North America.* 80(2): 729–744.

Welsby, PD, Richardson, A, Brettle, R.P. (1998). AIDS: Aspects in adults. In D. Doyle, G.W.C. Hanks, & N. MacDonald, Eds. *Oxford textbook of palliative medicine.* 2nd ed., (pp. 1121–1148). New York: Oxford University Press.

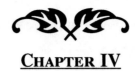

CHAPTER IV

PATIENT CARE: PAIN MANAGEMENT

Patricia Hinchliffe Berry, PhD, RN, CHPN, CS
Judith A. Paice, PHD, RN, FAAN

I. Introduction

A. Overview

1. Prevalence:

    a) Pain is experienced by 70 to 90 percent of patients with advanced disease, with 40–50% of patients experience moderate pain, and 25–30% have severe pain

    b) Pain scores (on a 0–10 scale) greater than or equal to "5" greatly impact on quality of life

2. It is estimated that almost all patients (85–90%) could be free of pain and 98–99% pain controlled using the knowledge and tools currently available; the remaining 1–2% of patients at end of life can be offered palliative sedation in addition to analgesics (defined as providing relief of refractory and intolerable symptoms with the use of sedatives at the end of life)

    a) This practice is within the realm of good supportive palliative care and is *not* euthanasia. The goal of sedation is to relieve distress from unrelenting physical, psychological or spiritual symptoms.

    b) This was formerly referred to as "terminal sedation", however this term led to confusion, suggesting assisted suicide, and the preferred terminology is palliative sedation

B. Barriers to both the assessment and the treatment of pain

1. Barriers from the patient/family perspective

    a) "Good" patients don't complain

    b) Pain is inevitable with aging

    c) Strong medicine only comes in injectable form

    d) Bearing the pain is better than bearing the side effects of pain medicine

e)   Addiction to pain medicine is common

f)   Strong pain medicine should only be used for very severe pain

g)   Morphine is a "last ditch drug" used only when one is imminently dying

2.   Barriers from the nurse and physician perspective

a)   The patient's self report of pain is not believed—health care professionals are the best judge of pain

b)   In the hospital setting, pain is often not seen as important as other indicators

c)   Only opioids are effective in severe pain

d)   Opioids cause respiratory depression

e)   Double effect (An ethical principle that permits an action, intended to have a good effect, when there is a risk of also causing a harmful effect, ONLY when the intention was to produce the good effect)

(1)   Double effect, as a principle guiding care, is complex, but nonetheless erroneously applied to end of life care, especially pain and symptom management

(2)   Adequately controlling symptoms at end of life is not known to shorten life

(3)   An analysis of the potential benefits of a therapy weighed against the possible risks should be conducted when considering any therapy

f)   The confusion over addiction/tolerance/physical dependence (see below)

g)   General lack of education relating to pain assessment, treatment, and pharmacology in basic and graduate education programs

(1)   There are still physicians and nurses who believe that morphine kills patients

(2)   There is a lack of knowledge regarding the treatment of chronic versus acute pain

3.   Other barriers that impact on reporting pain and using analgesics

a)   Anti-drug, "opio-phobic" culture—"Just say 'no' to drugs"

b)   Restrictions that vary by state, including triplicate prescription laws or other programs that monitor provider prescribing patterns, lack of laws facilitating pain management in end-stage illness, including partial filling of scheduled medications (fractioning)

C.   Important definitions

1.   *Pain:* Pain is whatever the experiencing person says it is, existing whenever he/she says it does[1]. History is 80% of the diagnosis—the patient's subjective report of pain is even more important to an accurate diagnosis, as there are no physical exam techniques or diagnostic tests to confirm pain history—***the patient's report must be accepted!***

2.   *Addiction:* Overwhelming involvement with obtaining and using a drug for its psychic benefits; not for medical reason; behavior is compulsive and subject to relapse; ***quality of life is not improved or enhanced; use continues despite harm***

3. *Tolerance:* After repeated administration of an opioid, a given dosage begins to lose its effectiveness; first in duration of action; second in overall effectiveness. Dose should be gradually titrated upward to maintain opioid's effectiveness

4. *Physical Dependence:* After repeated administration of an opioid, withdrawal symptoms occur when the drug is not taken

   a) Signs and symptoms of abstinence syndrome (withdrawal) include: anxiety, irritability, lacrimation, rhinorrhea, sweating, nausea, vomiting, cramps, insomnia, and *rarely* multifocal myoclonus

   b) Appearance of abstinence syndrome is a function of the elimination half-life of the opioid; for example, abstinence symptoms appear between 6–12 hours and peak between 24–72 hours following the last dose of a medication with a short half-life (morphine is an example)

   c) Conversely, with medications with a longer half-life, the appearance of abstinence symptoms are delayed, for example, with methadone, as much as 36 to 48 hours

5. Opioid *"pseudo-addiction:"* An iatrogenic syndrome in which patients develop certain behavioral characteristics of psychological dependence as a consequence of inadequate pain treatment[2]

II. **Assessment of Pain—effectiveness of pain management is directly related to assessment**

A. **Assessment parameters**

   1. *Site:* Have patient point on self or diagram, identify and assess all sites as well as sites of radiation; remember, also, the patient may have more than one site of pain; in that case, it would be helpful to number pains to organize assessment, interventions, and evaluations

   2. *Character:* Use the patient's *own* words; a careful description will lead to the diagnosis of pain type, and therefore use of appropriate adjuvant analgesics (i.e. sharp, shooting describes neuropathic pain syndromes); refer to the section, "Types of Pain," for additional, in depth descriptions

   3. *Onset:* When did it start? Did (or does) a specific event trigger the pain?

      a) Carefully distinguish between new and pre-existing pain (i.e. arthritis, chronic low back pain syndromes, etc.)

      b) Also assess for breakthrough pain

         (1) Transient flares of pain in patients with chronic pain syndromes are referred to as breakthrough pain

         (2) Breakthrough pain can be incidental (e.g., associated with movement), idiopathic (i.e., the cause is not known), or can occur as end-of-dose failure (e.g., the pain recurs prior to the next dose of pain medication)

   4. *Duration and frequency:* How long has the pain persisted? Is it constant or does it come and go (intermittent)?

5. *Intensity:* **Important note: ratings of pain intensity are the most important piece of pain assessment data to obtain if time is short; pain intensity directly correlates with interference with the patient's quality of life.**

   a) Commonly defined on a scale, most frequently 0-10, intensity rating

   b) Method must be adapted to patient.

   c) Record pain intensity "now," at its "worst," at its "least" and on an average.

   d) Pain rating scales for cognitively impaired or nonverbal patients are available, but caregivers (be they family or staff in a care facility) can often give valuable information to add to the pain assessment

      (1) A change in the patient's behavior, however, is considered the "gold standard"

      (2) One indicator of the presence of pain in patients who are unable to respond is the furrowed brow

      (3) Relief of the furrowing is often seen when pain is relieved; likewise, response to treatment can be considered part of the assessment

6. *Exacerbating factors:* What times, activities, or other circumstances make the pain worse?

7. *Associated symptoms:* What other symptoms occur before, with, or after the pain?

8. *Alleviating factors:* What makes the pain better? What treatments (including non-pharmacologic interventions) have been successful in the past and what have been unsuccessful? Include a thorough medication history

9. *Medication History:* What medications have been ordered? What medication is the patient currently taking? If there is a disparity, examine the underlying reasons (e.g., cost, adverse effects, fears of addiction or tolerance). What medications worked in the past for unrelated pain episodes? What are the patient/family/caregivers' beliefs about opioids?

10. *Impact on quality of life:* What does the pain mean to the patient and family? How has this pain affected them and their quality of life? Does it keep the patient from doing things he/she wants to do? How much do the patient and the family know about pain? Do they have the expectation that it can be relieved? Are there emotional or spiritual components to the pain? Does unrelieved pain lead to increased fear or anxiety, or to fears that death is imminent?

11. *Physical examination:* Observe the site of the pain, and validate with the patient the pain's location; note skin color, warmth, irritation, integrity and any other unusual findings; utilize other physical assessment techniques, for example, percussion and auscultation, as appropriate; be mindful that persons with chronic pain often have no changes in vital signs or facial expression.

B. Etiology of pain

1. Cancer Pain Syndromes

   a) Pain associated with direct tumor involvement

      (1) Direct tumor involvement accounts for approximately 78% of pain problems among cancer inpatients and 62% among cancer outpatients

      (2) Examples include metastatic bone disease, nerve compression or infiltration, hollow viscus involvement, among others

b) Pain associated with cancer therapy

    (1) Cancer therapy accounts for approximately 19% of pain problems among cancer inpatients and 25% among cancer outpatients

    (2) Examples include any pain that occurs in the course of or as a result of surgery, chemotherapy or radiation therapy (specific examples are mucositis, peripheral neuropathy, phantom pain syndromes, extravasation of vesicant chemotherapy)

c) Pain unrelated to cancer or cancer therapy

    (1) Incident pain accounts for approximately 3% of pain problems among cancer inpatients and 10% of pain problems among cancer outpatients

    (2) Examples include arthritis, osteoporosis, migraine headache, low back pain, fibromyalgia, or any other pain syndromes present among the general population

2. Pain syndromes common in the terminal phase of other medical conditions

a) HIV infection and AIDS

    (1) Statistics on the prevalence of pain in AIDS range from 30 to 97%, with an estimate of 50% relating directly to the HIV infection and 30% to the therapy for AIDS

    (2) HIV pain is often categorized in a manner similar to cancer: pain associated with the virus (e.g., direct involvement of the virus in the sensory neurons that transmit pain), pain associated with the treatment (e.g., neuropathy due to antiretroviral drugs), or pain unrelated to HIV or its treatment (e.g., musculoskeletal pains after exercise)

    (3) Examples of HIV/AIDS related pain include neuropathies (specifically peripheral neuropathy, acute and chronic polyneuropathy, symmetric distal sensory neuropathy, brachial plexopathy, herpetic neuralgia, cranial neuropathy, and headaches from acute and chronic meningitis), central pain from cerebral abscesses, esophagitis and abdominal pain from infectious gastrointestinal disease, chest pain from pneumocystis pneumonia, and generalized myalgias

b) Sickle cell disease

    (1) Three or more vascular occlusive episodes are a poor prognostic sign (less than 50% of those patients live beyond age 40). Hydroxyurea (Hydrea®) may decrease frequency of vaso-occlusive crises

    (2) Pain is severe and acute; focal (bone, joint and muscle) and visceral pain from ischemia and infarction

    (3) There are multiple myths and mistaken beliefs about sickle cell disease and sickle cell pain on the part of patients, their families, and the healthcare professions.

    (4) Factors related to race, ethnic, and class stereotyping in our culture further complicate this issue and serve as additional impediments to the control of pain in sickle cell disease[3]

    c)   Multiple sclerosis (MS)

        (1)   Pain is an issue in 55 to 82% of persons with MS

            (a)   Neurological (paroxysmal trigeminal neuralgia, optic neuritis and periorbital pain, extremity pain, including dysthesia, allodynia, and painful electric-shock sensations)

            (b)   Musculoskeletal (low back pain and extremity pain) in nature. Refer to Table 1 for definitions of the pain terms associated with neuropathic pain states

    d)   Cerebral vascular disease

        (1)   Post stroke pain is a problem in 1–2% of patients

            (a)   Often delayed for several years after the stroke; accompanied by decreased temperature sensation; may be superficial or deep; often severe in intensity and accompanied by hyperanalgesia and allodynia; may be elicited by emotional episodes and movement

            (b)   Another common post-stroke pain syndrome is mechanical shoulder pain unrelated to the central injury

    e)   Spinal cord injury: central pain may occur from an injury at any level of the spinal cord

C. Types of Pain

1. Acute pain: usually clear cause; meaningful; perceived as reversible; observable signs (such as increased pulse rate, increase in blood pressure; nonverbal signs and symptoms, such as facial expressions, tense muscles); examples: myocardial infarction, acute appendicitis

2. Chronic: often not a clear cause; does not fulfill a useful purpose; perceived as irreversible; cyclical (aching—agony); decreased social interaction, insomnia, depressed affect; few observable or behavioral signs; examples: cancer pain, chronic back pain

3. Nociceptive pain (or somatic and visceral pain) arises from direct stimulation of the afferent nerves due to tumor infiltration of skin, soft tissue, or viscera

    a)   Somatic pain: well-localized; often described as deep, dull ache; musculoskeletal in nature

        (1)   Examples: bone metastasis, inflammation of soft tissue, tumor invasion of soft tissue

        (2)   Can be controlled with conventional analgesics, (including NSAIDs if mild, and opioids, if moderate to severe) and in some cases, radiation therapy

    b)   Visceral pain: poorly localized; cramping, deep ache, pressure, often referred to distant dermatomal sites

        (1)   Examples: bowel obstruction, cholecystitis; metastatic tumors in the lung

        (2)   Can be controlled with conventional analgesics, and in some cases, antineoplastic treatments

4. Neuropathic pain results from actual injury to nerves rather than stimulation of nerve endings (Refer to Table 1 for definitions of pain terms associated with neuropathic pain states)

   a) Characteristics: sharp, burning, shooting, shock-like, sometimes associated with cyclovir and dysthesias (Refer to the table entitled Pain Terms Associated with Neuropathic Pain States)

   b) Examples: spinal nerve root compression, tumor invasion of nerves, post-herpetic neuralgia, surgical interruption of nerves, central pain syndromes occurring after stroke

   c) Response to conventional analgesics often poor (although this is controversial); but antidepressant, (e.g. nortriptyline) anticonvulsant (e.g. gabapentin, carbamazepine), corticosteroids and non-drug therapies may be beneficial as adjuvant analgesics to the opioids or in some cases as the primary analgesic.

5. Mixed nociceptive and neuropathic pain syndrome

   a) Common in life-threatening illnesses

   b) Thorough assessment is indicated

      (1) Pharmacological therapy is based upon these different pain syndromes

      (2) Occur concomitantly so patients may require agents from more than one category of analgesics (e.g., non-opioids, opioids, and adjuvants)

6. Referred pain is usually a visceral pain referred to skin, bone, and muscle, often distant from the site of origin

   a) Pain from tumor involvement of the pancreas, lower esophagus, stomach or retroperitoneal area may be referred to the back

   b) Gallbladder or liver disease may produce referred pain in the back or right shoulder (suprascapular)

   c) Rectosigmoid involvement may result in pain to sacrum or rectal area

D. **Factors that may influence the experience of pain:** Pain is experienced by the patient *and* family in keeping with the model of "total pain" and includes physical, psychological, social and spiritual effects; when adequate assessment and management of controllable symptoms precede psychological, social and spiritual assessment and intervention, overall outcomes often improve (Remember the lesson in Maslow's Hierarchy of needs); common effects of pain include:

1. Physical effects: Decreased functional ability, including ability to walk and perform other basic ADLs, decreased strength and endurance, nausea, anorexia, insomnia, and impaired immune response

2. Psychosocial effects: Alteration in social and close relationships, isolation, inability to work; loss of self-esteem, self-worth; increased caregiver burden, further disruption of important social supports for both patient and family

3. Emotional effects: Diminished leisure, increased fear and anxiety, depression, hopelessness, despair, loss of control; if pain uncontrolled, consideration of suicide or physician assisted suicide

4. Spiritual issues: Increased suffering, re-evaluation and perhaps doubt regarding past religious foundations and beliefs; questioning the meaning of suffering

5. Financial effects: Inability to work and earn income, loss of caregiver income, issues of workplace discrimination, and having to apply for governmental assistance leading to decreased income and loss of health insurance coverage

6. Cultural issues: Ethnic minority, female, and elderly persons often receive less than optimal pain management in all settings[4]

   a) Consider the patient's family of origin, their manner of expressing pain, and how suffering is valued

   b) Perceptions of pain, end of life, afterlife, bereavement and other aspects of palliative care vary widely by ethnicity and within ethnicities

   c) Be careful of "stereotyping," and do everything possible to learn about the patient and family's unique situation

   d) Specific aspects of culture to assess when caring for patients in pain include ethnic identity, gender, age, differing abilities, sexual orientation, religion and spirituality, financial status, place of residency, employment, and educational level

III. Pharmacologic Intervention*

A. Recommend medications according to severity and specific type of pain

1. World Health Organization (WHO) analgesic ladder

   a) Step one: mild pain (defined as a pain score of 1–4 on a 0–10 scale): non-opioids +/- adjuvants. Examples: aspirin, non-steroidal anti-inflammatory drug (NSAID), or acetaminophen (Tylenol®)

   b) Step two: moderate pain (defined as a pain score of 5–6 on a 0–10 scale): opioids +/- adjuvants. Examples: any opioid in smaller doses, codeine, hydrocodone (Vicodin®), oxycodone, morphine alone or in combination with a non-opioid

   c) Step three: severe pain (defined as a pain score of 7–10 on a 0–10 scale): opioids +/- adjuvants. Examples: morphine, hydromorphone (Dilaudid®), methadone, fentanyl (Duragesic®), oxycodone (Oxycontin®)

2. Drug actions and side effects

   a) Aspirin-like drugs (salicylates, and nonsalicylates [NSAIDs])

      (1) Actions: analgesic, antipyretic, anti-inflammatory, anti-thrombotic

      (2) Adverse effects

         (a) GI distress; no relation between symptoms and seriousness of GI effects; concomitant administration of misoprostol (Cytotec®) or omeprazole (Prilosec®) can prevent gastropathy

         (b) Renal insufficiency: elderly and dehydrated are at increased risk

         (c) Inhibiting of platelet aggregation

---

* Thanks to June L. Dahl, PhD, Professor of Pharmacology at the University of Wisconsin-Madison Medical School for her assistance with this section.

(d)   Hypersensitivity reactions (not allergic reactions); symptoms include urticaria, bronchospasm, severe rhinitis, and shock.

   (i)   Adverse effects are often labeled by patients/caregivers as "allergies" (e.g., nausea and vomiting)

   (ii)   These are not absolute contraindications to using the drug

(e)   CNS effects: dizziness, tinnitus, decreased hearing, headache

(3)   Dose escalation is limited by analgesic ceiling

b)   Acetaminophen (Tylenol®)

(1)   Actions: analgesic, antipyretic, *not anti-inflammatory*

(2)   Adverse effects: far fewer than with NSAIDs; hepatotoxic in large doses; ceiling is 4 grams a day, lower in alcoholic patients, AIDS patients, patients with liver metastasis or those with active liver disease. Dose escalation is limited by analgesic ceiling—consider quantity of acetaminophen in combination medications (Refer to table near the end of this section)

c)   Opioid medications

(1)   Pure agonists (morphine is prototype)

(2)   Mixed agonist-antagonists (pentazocine (Talwin®)), butorphanol (Stadol®), nalbuphine (Nubain®); *not recommended for the treatment of cancer pain due to analgesic ceiling, psychomimetic actions, precipitation of withdrawal when given to patients on opioids*

(3)   Action: bind to receptors in the brain, spinal cord and in periphery

(4)   Side effects of opioids:

(a)   Tolerance develops rapidly to the sedative, emetic, and respiratory depressant effects of opioids; however it does not develop to constipation

(b)   Sedation, sometimes, but rarely confusion

(c)   Dizziness, dysphoria

(d)   Nausea

(e)   Constipation; Tolerance *does not* develop—*must be prevented and treated aggressively*

(f)   Itching and urticaria

(g)   Respiratory depression

   (i)   Feared and misunderstood

   (ii)   Clinically significant respiratory depression is extremely rare when patients in severe pain receive opioids, especially in patients who are currently receiving opioids and when doses are titrated upward in appropriate steps; there are not good data to support the prevalence of respiratory depression due to opioids, however, there is general agreement that patients who are at risk are those who are opioid naïve and concomitantly taking other sedating drugs

(iii) Respiratory rate alone is not an indicator of respiratory depression; some patients may have a respiratory rate of 7, while alert and well perfused; other factors that must be considered are the level of sedation, the depth of respiration, and the adequacy of perfusion of oxygen in the tissues as determined by examining nail beds for changes in color, or obtaining an oxygen saturation level or pulse oximetry

(iv) How opioids cause respiratory depression: opioids render the CO_2 receptors gradually less sensitive to increasing CO_2 levels

(v) True respiratory depression (remember it is rare!) is best treated by slow infusion of *dilute* naloxone (Narcan®)

(5) Some other drug adverse effects include:

(a) Meperidine (Demerol®)

(i) Converted to a long-lived excitatory metabolite (normeperidine) causing shaky feelings, tremors/twitches, and myoclonus/grand mal seizures; should not be used in cancer pain management

(ii) Poor oral bioavailability

(b) Propoxyphene, the opioid in Darvon® and Darvocet® is, although widely prescribed, an

(i) Ineffective analgesic

(ii) Long-lived metabolite toxic to the central nervous system and cardiovascular system

(iii) Includes a large amount of acetaminophen. Therefore, it is not recommended for long-term use or use in the elderly

(c) Morphine

(i) Active metabolites (morphine 6-gluceronide, morphine 3-gluceronide), excreted by the kidneys that will be retained by elderly patients and by those with diminished renal function; has strong analgesic and respiratory depressant properties; M3G may produce central nervous system hyperexcitablilty and possibly myoclonus, while elevated M6G levels appear to cause sedation

(ii) Small amounts of hydration (IV fluids at 30–50cc/hr) helps to clear it through the kidneys

(iii) Hydromorphone (Dilaudid®) may be a safer choice for the elderly or those with diminished renal function

(6) No dosage ceiling for most opioids—so are able to titrate to effect (Important note: codeine, hydrocodone, cyclovir and all mixed agonist/antagonists do have dosage ceilings and thus, cannot be titrated to effect)

(7) Choosing delivery routes

    (a) Oral: most preferred for comfort, convenience, and cost effectiveness; many forms available, immediate release tablets, sustained release tablets, liquids; Oralettes are now available as well. Sublingual is same as oral route however differs from the transdermal route

    (b) Rectal: useful for patients who are NPO or have nausea and vomiting; contraindicated with anal lesions, diarrhea, constipation, or leukopenia; varying comfort levels with family caregivers and some cultures

    (c) Subcutaneous or intravenous infusion: rarely required, but useful for pain requiring rapid titration of medication; while subcutaneous infusion is useful in most cases, impaired circulation or the presence of fibrosis can compromise absorption; used extensively at home for patients who are obstructed or who can no longer swallow and have severe pain. Can be managed within home setting; especially useful if parenteral route required and reliable or intravenous access not possible. Expense of home parenteral infusions to hospice programs are a barrier to use

    (d) Intramuscular injections should be avoided, injections are painful, unnecessary and absorption is not reliable

    (e) Transmucosal: easily accessible route, provides rapid onset of action and is much faster if used with lipophilic drugs such as fentanyl

    (f) Transdermal (e.g. fentanyl [Duragesic®]) for patients with stable pain (not good for rapid titration of medication); reservoir in subcutaneous tissue, delayed onset of action (12–24 hours), so patient must have an immediate release medication during the first several hours after the fentanyl patch is applied, some patients require a patch change every 48 hours; should not be given to opioid naïve patients

    (g) Spinal: via indwelling catheters into the epidural or intrathecal space; an implantable pump should be used in only carefully selected patients after appropriate consultation; cost, care issues, and potential adverse effects should also be carefully weighed however can dramatically improve some patients quality of life especially with severe pain in lower extremities

d) Adjuvant analgesics

    (1) For treatment of neuropathic pain

        (a) Tricyclic antidepressants

            (i) Desipramine (Norpramin®) and nortriptyline (Pamelor®)recommended over amitryiptyline, which has more anticholinergic effects (causing cardiovascular changes, dry mouth, constipation)

            (ii) Serotonin selective reuptake inhibitors (SSRI's) have not been well studied in neuropathic pain and may seem to have limited analgesic effect.

            (iii) Guidelines for use

                (a) Start with a low dose (e.g., desipramine 25 mg po or nortriptyline 10–25 mg at bedtime (these drugs may cause sedation and enhance sleep)

(b) Increase dose by 10–25 mg increments every few days based upon the patient's response

(c) Response may be delayed by 3–7 days

(d) Monitor adverse effects

(e) Maximum dose of nortriptyline and desipramine is 300 mg/day

(f) Adverse effects: sedation, orthostatic hypotension, anticholinergic side effects (including urinary retention), cardiac effects

(b) Anticonvulsants

(i) Most useful for lancinating, paroxysmal pain and pain that doesn't respond to antidepressant therapy; dose as with seizures; most experience has been with carbamazepine

(ii) Gabapentin (300–1800 mg TID); Carbamazepine (100–800 mg BID or QID); Phenytoin (100–200 mg TID); Valproic acid (200–400 mg BID or TID); Clonazepam (0.25–.5 mg TID); (All doses are P.O.)

(iii) Guidelines for use:

(a) Start low, go slow

(b) Watch for side effects

(c) Monitor serum levels for signs of toxicity

(iv) Major adverse effects:

(a) Gabapentin (Neurontin®): sedation, side effects generally less than with others (has less bone marrow suppression—drug of choice for patients on chemotherapy); costly

(b) Carbamazepine (Tegretol®): bone marrow suppression, vertigo, confusion, sedation

(c) Phenytoin (Dilantin®): ataxia, rash, hepatotoxicity

(d) Valproic acid (Depakene®): nausea, vomiting, sedation, ataxia, tremor, thrombocytopenia, neutropenia, hepatotoxicity

(e) Clonazepam (Klonopin®): sedation, physical dependence

(c) Local anesthetics

(i) Useful in refractory neuropathic pain

(ii) Lidocaine, given IV (more likely to be offered outside hospice program); tocainide (Tonocard®) and mexiletine (Mexitil®), given orally

(iii) Adverse effects include dizziness, lightheadedness, lowered blood pressure, sensory disturbances and tremor, seizures at high doses, nausea and vomiting

(iv) Lidocaine 5% is also available in a patch for topical relief of postherpetic neuropathy, post-thoracotomy pain and other pain syndromes

(a) The patches should be placed over intact skin only

(b) Up to three patches can be used to cover the painful area and are left in place for 12 hours, with 12 hours off

(c) Adverse effects are uncommon and include pain with removal of the patch

(d) Patients with sensitivity to touch (also called allodynia) often report relief

(d) Baclofen (Lioresal®) (muscle relaxant): used to treat a variety of neuropathic pain problems

(2) Corticosteroids: used in metastatic bone pain (triple effect of pain control, mood elevation and increased appetite)

(3) Topical capsaicin (Zostrix®): used for diabetic neuropathy, postherpetic neuralgia, arthritis, Kaposi's Sarcoma lesions

(4) Other medications used to treat side effects of opioids e.g. psychostimulants, phenothiazines, benzodiazepines (muscle spasms)

3. Opioid Equianalgesic conversions

a) Process

(1) Step 1. Add up the total amount of the current drug given in 24 hours; remember to add in both the scheduled and breakthrough or rescue doses; calculate separately if more than one drug used

(2) Step 2. Divide current 24-hour total by the equianalgesic value for the current drug and route of administration (see chart on page 161)

(3) Step 3. Multiply the above number by the equianalgesic value for the new drug and route; this will give you the new 24-hour dose

(4) Step 4. Determine how many doses the patient will take each day and divide this number into the total 24-hour dose; this gives the amount of medication needed per dose

b) Example:

(1) The patient is taking 2 tablets of acetaminophen in combination with hydrocodone 5mg every 4 hours. Because each tablet contains 5 mg of hydrocodone, two contain 10 mg. 6 doses x 10mg = 60 mg/day of hydrocodone; convert to oral hydromorphone

(2) 60mg of hydrocodone divided by 30 mg (equivalent value for hydrocodone) = 2

(3) 2 x 7.5mg (equivalent value for oral hydromorphone) = 15mg (or 15mg of hydromorphone in 24 hours)

(4) Hydromorphone can be given every 4 hours, which is 6 doses a day; divide the 24 hour dose by 6 doses; *(15 divided by 6 = 2.5)* **2.5 mg hydromorphone every 4 hours;** since hydromorphone comes in 2, 4, and 8 mg tablets, round the dose down to 2 mg, order appropriate breakthrough medications, and carefully monitor the patient for the need to increase the dose

4. Calculating breakthrough or rescue doses

    a) A rescue dose is always ordered with long-acting opioids; it is preferable to match the breakthrough medication with the long-acting opioid, e.g., immediate release morphine with sustained release morphine

    b) Doses should increase commensurate with increases in the scheduled doses

    c) The 1999 the American Pain Society guidelines recommend using 10–15% of the 24-hour oral dose, given every 2 hours as needed

    d) Other clinical reports suggest the breakthrough dose should be 10–20% of the 24-hour dose and since the peak effect is usually within one hour, doses can be repeated every hour

    e) For parenteral administration (IV or SQ), the breakthrough dose is 50–100% of the hourly rate; since the peak effect is in 15 minutes, boluses may be given safely in the majority of patients every 15 minutes

    f) Increase baseline dose of long-acting opioid if more than 3 rescue doses are used in 24 hours

    g) Example: a patient is taking 120 mg MS Contin (long acting morphine) every 12 hours; the appropriate breakthrough dose of MSIR (immediate release morphine) is 24–36 mg (10–15%) every 2 hours as needed

B. **Nonpharmacologic interventions can be used concurrently with medications and other modalities to relieve pain and can often be taught to patients and/or family members; there are some that believe that medications should never be given without the addition of** *some* **nonpharmacologic intervention. However, the use of nonpharmacologic interventions should** *never* **preclude appropriate use of medications, including opioids. The most common nonpharmacologic interventions are listed below:**

1. Physical modalities

    a) Consider PT and OT consults (especially in the inpatient palliative care setting)

    b) Cutaneous stimulation (heat, cold)

    c) Exercise (with limitations based on physical condition)

    d) Transcutaneous nerve stimulation (efficacy controversial may be useful in patients with mild pain); acupuncture

    e) Massage; healing touch; therapeutic touch

2. Psychosocial and spiritual interventions (helpful in maintaining control in uncertain, dependent, and anxiety-provoking situations)

    a) Relaxation and guided imagery

    b) Distraction

        c)   Music

        d)   Reframing

        e)   Patient/family education

        f)   Hypnosis

        g)   Counseling

        h)   Prayer

        i)   Spiritual reflection or meditation

3.   Other

        a)   Biofeedback

        b)   Aromatherapy

4.   Palliative radiation therapy

        a)   May be used to relieve symptoms of patients with advanced disease, (e.g., pain, bleeding), compression of vital organ systems, (e.g., the brain, ulcerating skin lesions), and metastasis to weight bearing bones susceptible to fracture

        b)   Radiation therapy is the treatment of choice for spinal cord compression, bone pain and is frequently used in superior vena cava syndrome and symptomatic brain metastases

        c)   While external beam radiation is the modality commonly used for palliative radiation therapy, Strontium-89, an intravenous radionucleotide that emits beta radiation at the bony metastatic site, is sometimes used to treat areas of painful skeletal metastasis; newer radionucleotides are currently under study that may not produce the painful flair that occurs when Strontium-89 is given

5.   Palliative chemotherapy: may improve or enhance comfort when neither cure nor control is possible

        a)   Antineoplastic therapy may produce tumor shrinkage, relief of pressure on nerves, lymphatics, and blood vessels and reduction in organ obstruction, thus relieving pain

        b)   Bisphosphonates are useful in treating pain related to multiple myeloma and metastatic bone disease[5]

IV. Pain During the Final Days of Life

A. Pain assessment

1.   Patients may become nonverbal in the final days of life

        a)   A furrowed brow may indicate pain

        b)   Guarding and vocalization during turning or dressing changes may suggest pain

        c)   A therapeutic trial of an opioid should be strongly considered to determine if these behaviors change with the use of an analgesic

2.   If the patient had pain prior to becoming unresponsive, assume pain is still present

B. Pharmacologic management

1. As organ system dysfunction increases, particularly renal clearance, drugs or their metabolites are cleared from the body less efficiently and sedation may increase

   a) Therefore, a therapeutic trial of opioid dose reduction may be indicated if sedation is not a desired effect

   b) In some cases, patients may become more alert and responsive

   c) If any signs of pain return, the dose should be returned to its previous level

2. Rapid discontinuation of opioids, benzodiazepines or other agents can result in the abstinence syndrome; whenever possible, gradual reduction in dose of these drugs is indicated

3. Sedation at the end of life is an option for patients with intractable pain and suffering[5]

   a) There are numerous combinations of medications that are used to accomplish sedation

      (1) Opioids

      (2) Barbiturates

      (3) Neuroleptics

      (4) Benzodiazepines

   b) Therapy is based on obtaining initial relief of symptoms followed by ongoing sedation to maintain the effect

   c) Parenteral ketamine, given either as a continuous infusion or as bolus doses, may also be used to accomplish sedation at the end of life

C. Nonpharmacologic management should continue

V. Summary of Principles of Pain Managment

A. Pain assessment data is documented so the pain etiology or syndrome can be identified and appropriately treated

B. The oral route is used whenever possible

1. If the patient is unable to take PO medications, buccal, sublingual, rectal, and transdermal routes are considered before parenteral routes

2. IM route is avoided

3. IV and subcutaneous route can be used for any patient that cannot tolerate above choices under oral route or when pain is rapidly escalating and severe. Subcutaneous route is a useful alternative in the home setting when reliable IV access is not possible

C. **Constant pain calls for treatment with an around-the-clock scheduled long acting opioid and a short acting medication for breakthrough pain**

1. Only one long-acting opioid is ordered for constant pain

2. Doses of opioids are increased commensurate with the patient's report of pain

3. Equianalgesic conversions are used when changing medications and/or routes

4. Adjuvant medications are used for neuropathic pain, some visceral pain states, and bone pain

D. **Breakthrough pain**

1. Only one analgesic is ordered for breakthrough pain

2. Use an adequate rescue dose for breakthrough pain; American Pain Society (APS) rescue dose recommendation is 10–15% of the 24-hour dose q2h PRN; always increase the rescue dose when the baseline dose is increased

3. Increase the baseline dose if the patient needs more than 3 rescue doses in 24 hours unless pain is related to a specific activity or if patient becomes sedated with increased around the clock dose

4. A higher dosage of breakthrough, or rescue medication, is sometimes necessary if the frequency of breakthrough pain and/or intensity are at higher levels

5. To calculate rescue dose when fentanyl (Duragesic®) is used, divide the total patch dose by 3—that is the appropriate dose of MSIR; (immediate release morphine). All chronic pain requires the use of breakthrough pain medication

6. Patients and families need to be educated about taking the medication when the pain is first perceived—not when it has become severe or unbearable

E. **Non-pharmacologic approaches are always a part of any pain management plan**

F. **An appropriate preventative bowel regimen is ordered with a stimulant laxative and stool softener to correct the effects of the opioid. Refer to the chapter on symptom management**

VI. **Evaluation—pain management is predicated by ongoing assessment of treatment efficacy and control of treatment side effects.**

A. **Evaluation of interventions is a basic nursing function and completes the nursing process**

B. **Nursing evaluation should be accomplished in a timely manner, in accordance with expected pharmacologic peak action or when the non-pharmacologic intervention is completed**

C. **At each nursing visit assess for:**

1. Pain intensity, type, duration, etc.

2. Medication side effects, interactions or complications

3. Patient's satisfaction with method of pain relief

D. In the in-patient setting

1. Pain assessment every shift or more frequently as indicated

2. Patient/family teaching and reinforcement of pain management

3. Monitor bowel status daily and document

E. Evaluate efficacy of pain relief interventions with a thorough assessment

1. At appropriate intervals after any change in medication, dosage, route of administration, etc.

2. At each nursing visit

Table 1: Opioid Dosing Equivalence

Drug	Dose (mg) Parenteral	Dose (mg) Oral	Duration (hours)
Morphine (IR)	10	30	3–4
Morphine, Controlled Release (MS Contin®, Oramorph SR®)	—	30	8–12
Hydromorphone (Dilaudid®)	1.5	7.5	3–4
Codeine	130	200	3–4
Oxycodone, Controlled Release (Oxycontin®)	—	20–30	8–12
Oxycodone (Roxicodone® Percocet®)	—	20–30	3–4
Hydrocodone (Vicodin®; Lortab®)	—	30	3–4
Meperidine (Demerol®)[2]	100	300+	2–3
Levorphenol (Levo-dromoran®)	2	4	6–8
Methadone (Dolophine®)[3] (Paice & Fine, 2001)	10 acute pain 2–4 chronic pain	20 acute pain 2–4 chronic pain	6–8
Fentanyl (Duragesic®)	0.1	Convert present medication to 24 hour oral MS equivalent; then divide in half; this is mcg/hr dose of Fentanyl	48–72
Propoxyphene (Darvon®; Darvocet®)[4]	—	180	4

---

[2] WARNING: Long-lived toxic metabolite; CNS stimulant, not recommended for long-term use

[3] Methadone to morphine oral equipotent ratio may be closer to 10 to 1 rather than 3 to 2; caution is advised. A good review of the use of Methadone is given in the reference list (Ripamonti, C., Zecca, E. & Bruera, E., 1997)

[4] WARNING: Long-lived metabolite that is toxic to the central nervous system and cardiovascular system, not recommended for long-term use and use in the elderly.

Table 2: Combination Products

Opioid	Proprietary name and combination drugs[6]
Hydrocodone	Vicodin® (5mg + 500mg acetaminophen) Vicodin ES® (7.5mg + 750mg acetaminophen) Lorcet-10® (10mg + 650mg acetaminophen) Lortab® Vicodin HP® (10mg + 660mg acetaminophen) Norco® (10mg + 325mg acetaminophen) Anexsia® (5mg + 500mg acetaminophen) Zydone® (5mg + 400mg acetaminophen)
Oxycodone	Percodan® (5mg + 325mg ASA) Percocet® (5mg + 325mg acetaminophen) Tylox® (5mg + 500mg acetaminophen) Roxicet® (5mg + 325mg acetaminophen)
Codeine	Tylenol #2® (15mg + 325mg acetaminophen) Tylenol #3® (30mg + 325mg acetaminophen) Tylenol #4® (60mg + 325mg acetaminophen)
Propoxyphene[5]	Darvon® (65mg) Darvocet N® (100mg + 650mg acetaminophen) Darvon Compound® (65mg + 325mg ASA + caffeine) Darvon-N® or Darvon©® with ASA (65mg + 325mg ASA)

[5] WARNING: Long-lived metabolite that is toxic to the central nervous system and cardiovascular system, not recommended for long-term use and use in the elderly.

[6] Twenty-four hour dose of acetaminophen should not exceed 4 grams for adults

Table 3: Pain Terms Associated With Neuropathic Pain States (modified from the International Association for the Study of Pain; McCaffery and Pasero)

Term	Definition
Allodynia	Pain due to a stimulus, which does not normally provoke pain
Dysesthesia	An unpleasant abnormal sensation, whether spontaneous or evoked
Hyperalgesia	A painful syndrome characterized by an abnormally painful reaction to a normally non-painful stimulus, such as touch. (Sometimes referred hyperpathia)
Paresthesia	An abnormal anesthetic sensation (often described as a painful numbness)
Neuralgia	Pain in the distribution of a nerve or nerves
Neuropathic pain	Pain initiated or caused by a primary lesion or dysfunction in the nervous system
Peripheral neuropathic pain	Pain initiated or caused by a primary lesion or dysfunction in the peripheral nervous system (e.g., postherpetic neuropathy).
Central pain	Pain initiated or caused by a primary lesion or dysfunction in the central nervous system. (e.g., post-thalamic pain syndrome occurring after stroke)

References

1. McCaffery, M. and C. Pasero, *Pain: Clinical Manual.* 1999, St. Louis, MO: Mosby.

2. Weissman, D.E., J.L. Dahl, and P.A. Dinndorf, *Handbook of cancer pain management.* 1996, Madison, WI: The Wisconsin Cancer Pain Initiative.

3. Benjamin, L.J., et al., *Guideline for the Management of Acute and Chronic Pain in Sickle-Cell Disease.* 1999, Skokie, IL: American Pain Society.

4. Cleelan, C., et al., *Pain and its treatment in outpatients with metastatic cancer.* New England Journal of Medicine, 1994. **330:** p. 592–596.

5. Paice, J.A. and P. Fine, *Pain at the end of life, in Textbook of palliative nursing,* B. Ferrell and N. Coyle, Editors. 2001, Oxford University Press: New York. p. 76–90.

General References

American Geriatric Society Panel on Chronic Pain in Older Persons. (1998). The management of chronic pain in older persons. *Journal of the American Geriatrics Society,* 46, 635–651.

American Medical Directors Association. (1999). *Chronic Pain Management in the Long-Term Care Setting.* Columbia, MD: Author.

American Pain Society. (1999). *Principles of analgesic use in the treatment of acute pain and cancer pain, (3rd Ed).* Skokie, IL. Author.

American Pain Society Quality of Care Committee. (1995). Quality improvement guidelines for the treatment of acute pain and cancer pain. *JAMA,* 23, 1874–1880.

Berry, P. & Ward, S. E. (1995). Caregiver-related barriers to adequate pain management in hospice. *Hospice Journal,* 10(4), 19–33.

Berry, P., Zeri, K. and Egan, K. (1997). *The hospice nurses study guide: A preparation for the CRNH candidate, (2nd ed.).* Pittsburgh, PA: Hospice Nurses Association.

Carr DB, Jacox A, Chapman CR, et al. (1992). *Acute Pain Management: Operative or Medical Procedures and Trauma: Clinical Practice Guideline No. 1.* Rockville, MD US Public Health Service, Agency for Health Care Policy and Research; AHCPR publication 92–0032.

Coluzzi, P., Volker, B. and Miaskowski, C. (Eds.). (1996). *Comprehensive pain management in terminal illness.* Sacramento, CA: California State Hospice Association.

Cunningham, M.L., Ruger, T.F., & Thorpe, D.M., (Eds.). (1998). *M.D. Anderson cancer center nursing reports on strategies for pain management; Assessment of pain syndromes in cancer patients.* Newtown PA; Associates in Medical Marketing.

Doyle, D., Hanks, G.W.C. and MacDonald, N. (Eds.). (1998). *The oxford textbook of palliative medicine. (2nd ed.).* New York: Oxford University Press.

Enck, R. (1994). *The medical care of terminally ill patients.* Baltimore: Johns Hopkins University Press.

Ersek, M. & Ferrell, B. R. (1994). Providing relief from cancer pain by assisting in the search for meaning. *Journal of Palliative Care,* 10(4), 15–22.

Ewald, G.A. and McKenzie, C.R. (Eds.). (1995). *Manual of medical therapeutics: The Washington manual.* St. Louis, MO: Department of Medicine, Washington University.

Federation of State Medical Boards of the United States, Inc. (1998). *Model Guidelines for the Use of Controlled Substances for the Treatment of Pain.* Euless, TX: author.

Ferrell, B.R. (Ed.). (1996). *Suffering.* Sudbury, MA: Jones and Bartlett.

Ferrell, B. R., Cohen, M. Z., Rhiner, M., & Rozek, A. (1991). Pain as a metaphor for illness: Part II: Family caregivers management of pain. *Oncology Nursing Forum,* 18, 1315–1321.

Ferrell, B. R. & Dean, G. (1995). The meaning of cancer pain. *Seminars in Oncology Nursing,* 11(1), 17–22.

Ferrell, B. R., Rhiner, M., Cohen, M. Z., & Grant, M. (1991). Pain as a metaphor for illness: Part I: Impact of pain on family caregivers. *Oncology Nursing Forum,* 18, 1303–1309.

Ferrell, B. R., Taylor, E. J., Grant, M., Fowler, M., Corbisiero, R. M., (1993). Pain management at home: struggle, comfort and mission. *Cancer Nursing,* 16, 169–178.

Ferrell, B. R., Taylor, E. J., Sattler, G. R., Fowler, M., & Cheyney, B. L. (1993). Searching for the meaning of pain. *Cancer Practice,* 1(3), 185–193.

Flaskerud, J., & Ungvarski, P. (1992). *HIV/AIDS: A guide to nursing care, (2nd ed.).* Philadelphia: W.B. Saunders.

Foley, G., Fochtman, D., & Mooney, K. (Eds.). (1993.) *Nursing care of the child with cancer. (2nd ed.).* Philadelphia: W.B. Saunders.

Foley, K.M. (1998). Pain assessment and cancer pain syndromes. In Doyle, D., Hanks, G.W.C. and MacDonald, N. (Eds.). *Oxford textbook of palliative medicine, (2nd ed.).* (pp. 310–331). New York: Oxford University Press.

Griffie, J., Muchka, S., Matson, S., & Weissman, D.E. (1998). *Improving Pain Management in Long Term Care Settings,* Milwaukee, WI: Palliative Care Program, Medical College of Wisconsin. (available from: www.mcw.edu/pallmed/)

Griffie, J., Muchka, S., & Weissman, D.E. (2000). *Nursing Staff Education Resource Manual: Pain Management 101.* Milwaukee, WI: Palliative Care Program, Medical College of Wisconsin. (available from:www.mcw.edu/palmed/)

Gordon, D. B., Dahl, J. L., Stevenson, K. K. (2000). *Building an Institutional Commitment to Pain Management: The Wisconsin Resource Manual (2nd ed.),* Madison: University of Wisconsin-Madison Board of Regents.

Hanks, G., Portenoy, R.K., Macdonald, N. and Forbes, K. (1998). Difficult pain problems. In Doyle, D., Hanks, G.W.C. and MacDonald, N. (Eds.). *Oxford textbook of palliative medicine, (2nd ed.).* (pp. 454–477). New York: Oxford University Press.

Jacox A, Carr DB, Payne R, et al. (1994). *Management of Cancer Pain: Adults: Clinical Practice Guideline No. 9.* Rockville, MD US Public Health Service, Agency for Health Care Policy and Research; AHCPR publication 94–0593.

Johanson, G. (1994). *Physician handbook of symptom relief in terminal care (4th ed.).* Santa Rosa, CA: Sonoma County Academic Foundation for Excellence in Medicine, (http://www.members.aol.com/scafem).

Kaye, P. (1995). *Notes on symptom control in hospice and palliative care.* Essex, CT: Hospice Education Institute. (1-800-544-2213).

Kovach, C., Weissman, D.E., Griffie, J., Matson, S., & Muchka, S. (1999). Assessment and treatment of discomfort for people with late-stage dementia. *Journal of Pain and Symptom Management,* 18, 412–419.

Kovach, C., Griffie, J., Muchka, S, Noonan, P., & Weissman, D.E. (2000). Nurses' perceptions of pain assessment and treatment in cognitively impaired elderly. *Clinical Nurse Specialist,* 14, 215–220.

Levy, M.H. (1996). Pharmacologic treatment of cancer pain. *New England Journal of Medicine,* 335, 1124–1132.

Marzinski, L. R. (1991). The tragedy of dementia: Clinically assessing pain in the confused, nonverbal elderly. *Journal of Gerontological Nursing,* 17 (6), 25–28.

Mather, L.E. (1994). The clinical effects of morphine pharmacology. *Regional Anesthesia,* 20(4), 263–282.

McGuire, D.B., Yarbro, C.H., & Ferrell, B.R. (1995). *Cancer pain management (2nd ed.).* Boston: Jones and Bartlett.

Mount, B. (1993). Whole person care: Beyond psychosocial & physical needs. *American Journal of Hospice & Palliative Care,* 10(1), 28–37.

Payne, R. and Gonzales, G.R. (1998). Pathophysiology of pain in cancer and other terminal diseases. In Doyle, D., Hanks, G.W.C. and MacDonald, N. (Eds.). *Oxford textbook of palliative medicine, (2nd. Ed.).* (pp. 299–310). New York: Oxford University Press.

Portenoy, R.K. (1995). Pharmacologic management of cancer pain. *Seminars in Oncology,* 22(2), suppl. 3 (April), pp. 112–120.

Portenoy, R. K. (1989). Cancer pain: Epidemiology and syndromes. *Cancer,* 63, 2298–2307.

Ripamonti, C., Zecca, E. & Bruera, E. (1997). An update on the clinical use of methadone for cancer pain. *Pain,* 70, 109–115.

Serlin, R. C., Mendoza, T. R., Nakamura, Y., Edwards, K. R., & Cleeland, C. S. (1995). When is cancer pain mild, moderate or severe? Grading pain severity by its interference with function. *Pain,* 61, 277–284.

Spross, J., McGuire, D.B. Schmitt, R.M. (1990). Oncology Nursing Society position paper on cancer pain. Part I, *Oncology Nursing Forum,* 17(5), 595–614.

Storey, P. and Knight, C.F. (1996 & 1997). *Hospice/Palliative care training for physicians.* (UNIPACS 2,3,4,6). Gainesville, FL: American Academy of Hospice and Palliative Medicine. (http://www.aahpm@aahpm.org).

SUPPORT Study Principle Investigators. (1995). A controlled trial to improve care for seriously ill hospitalized patients: A study to understand prognoses and preferences for outcomes and risks of treatments (SUPPORT). *Journal of the American Medical Association,* 274, 1591–1598.

Turk, D., & Feldman, C. (Eds.). (1992). Noninvasive approaches to pain management in the terminally ill. *Hospice Journal,* 8(1/2), entire issue.

U. S. Department of Health and Human Services. (1992). *Clinical practice guideline: Acute pain management: Operative or medical procedures.* (AHCPR publication No. 92–0032). Washington, DC: Government Printing Office.

U. S. Department of Health and Human Services. (1994). *Clinical practice guideline: Management of cancer pain.* (AHCPR Publication No. 94–0592). Washington, DC: U.S. Government Printing Office. (AHCPR Web Site: http://www.ahcpr.gov; 1-800-358-9295).

Volker, B.G. (Ed.). (1999). *Hospice and Palliative Nurses Practice Review, (3rd ed.).* Dubuque, Iowa: Kendall/Hunt.

Von Roenn, J. H., Cleeland, C. S., Gonin, R., Hatfield, A. K., & Pandya, K. J. (1993). Physician attitudes and practice in cancer pain management. *Annals of Internal Medicine,* 119, 121–126.

Ward, S. E., Berry, P., & Misiewicz, H. (1996). Concerns about analgesics among patient and family caregivers in a hospice. *Research in Nursing and Health,* 19, 205–211.

Ward, S. E., Goldberg, N., Miller-McCauley, V., Mueller, C., Nolan, A., Pawlik-Plank, D., Robbons, A., Stormoen, D., & Weissman, D. E. (1993). Patient-related barriers to management of cancer pain. *Pain,* 52, 319–324.

Weissman, D.E., Griffie, J., Muchka, S., Matson, S. (2000). Building an institutional commitment to pain management in long term care facilities. *Journal of Pain and Symptom Management,* 20, 35–43.

Wrede-Seaman, L. (1999). *Symptom management algorithms: A handbook for palliative care, (2nd ed.).* Yakima, WA: Intellicard.

World Health Organization. (1990). *Cancer pain relief.* Geneva, Switzerland.

Zeri, K., Egan, K, & Shubert, V. (1994). *Hospice nurses certification exam review: A self-study guide.* Pittsburgh: Hospice Nurses Association.

CHAPTER V

SYMPTOM MANAGEMENT

Cathleen A. Collins, RN, MSN, CHPN
Margery A. Wilson, MSN, FNP, CHPN

I. **Principles**

    A.   **The nursing process (using assessment, diagnosis, planning, for symptom management and care at the end-of-life)**

    B.   **Care at the end-of-life is multidimensional with emphasis on quality-of-life as the patient and family define it, with respect for, support and education of patient and family**

    C.   **Understanding of expectations, goals of treatment, end-of-life goals. Issues must be clarified with patient and family, taking into account the patient's position on the disease trajectory**

    D.   **The interdisciplinary team (IDT) is the framework for palliative care and hospice**

    E.   **The patient and family are the unit of care in palliative care and hospice and are included in the assessment, planning, decision-making and evaluation of interventions**

        1.   Options and expected or possible outcomes are discussed with patient and family to inform their decision-making; the IDT is responsible for giving them information regarding the benefits and the burdens of any treatment that is proposed

        2.   Patients and families require time, opportunity for clarification and review in anticipation of making decisions

    F.   **The end-of-life can be a time of growth, reconciliation, peace, joy and hope for patients and families; appropriate symptom management can facilitate this process by maximizing patient comfort**

    G.   **Authors' note: Patients may experience a variety of symptoms. Those covered in this chapter are some of the most often experienced by individuals with life-threatening illness**

II.   Alteration in Skin and Mucous Membranes

    A.   Definition: disruption in the integrity of the skin or oral mucous membrane

    B.   Possible etiologies

        1.   Skin integrity

            a)   Pressure ulcers

                (1)   Pressure to the skin, causing a decrease in blood flow and eventual cell death

                (2)   Shearing forces, in which two surfaces slide in opposite but parallel directions (e.g., a patient slides down in bed and bone and skin are displaced from one another)

                (3)   Friction, in which two surfaces move across one another (e.g., patient is dragged across bed sheets)

                (4)   Moisture (especially feces and urine)

                (5)   Obesity

                (6)   Malnutrition

                (7)   Immobility

                (8)   Impaired circulation due to peripheral vascular disease, diabetes, or cancer infiltration through skin

            b)   Fistulas

            c)   Tumor necrosis

        2.   Alteration of oral mucous membranes

            a)   Dry mouth (xerostomia)

                (1)   Candidiasis

                (2)   Drugs (anticholinergics, antihistamines, phenothiazines)

                (3)   Radiation and chemotherapy

                (4)   Dehydration

                (5)   Mucositis

                (6)   Mouth breathing

                (7)   Metabolic disorders (hypercalcemia, hyperglycemia)

            b)   Candidiasis

                (1)   Radiation and chemotherapy

                (2)   Drugs (antibiotics, corticosteroids)

            c)   Herpes simplex virus

            d)   Mucositis caused by radiation or chemotherapy

3.   Pruritis: uncomfortable itching of the skin

    a)   Dry, flaky skin

    b)   Wet, macerated skin

    c)   Contact dermatitis caused by ointments or creams

    d)   Infestations caused by scabies, lice, fleas

    e)   Drugs (antibiotics, morphine, phenothiazines)

    f)   Systemic disease (renal failure, hepatobiliary disease, infiltration of tumors into subcutaneous tissue)

    g)   Fungal infections

C.   Assess for:

1.   Skin integrity

    a)   Inspect skin each time patient changes position

    b)   If pressure ulcer, grade wound according to stage[1]

        (1)   Stage I: Nonblanchable erythema of intact skin, the heralding lesion of skin ulceration

            (a)   In individuals with dark skin, discoloration of the skin, warmth, edema, induration, or hardness also may be indicators

            (b)   Skin changes may be difficult to discern in some persons of color and the patient's report of pain may be the only clue to closely examine at-risk areas; be mindful of baseline skin color and monitor skin frequently for skin color change

        (2)   Stage II: Partial thickness skin loss involving epidermis, dermis, or both. The ulcer is superficial and presents clinically as an abrasion, blister, or shallow crater

        (3)   Stage III: Full thickness skin loss involving damage to or necrosis of subcutaneous tissue that may extend down to, but not through, underlying fascia. The ulcer presents clinically as a deep crater with or without undermining of adjacent tissue

        (4)   Stage IV: Full thickness skin loss with extensive destruction, tissue necrosis, or damage to muscle, bone, or supporting structures; undermining and sinus tracts also may be associated with Stage IV pressure ulcers

    c)   Wound location

    d)   Wound appearance

        (1)   Size, length, width, depth, undermining

        (2)   Presence of drainage (serous, serosanguineous, sanguineous, purulent)and amount

        (3)   Tissue type (i.e., granulating or eschar)

        (4)   Appearance of surrounding skin (redness, maceration, etc.)

e) Is wound painful?

f) If wound is due to tumor necrosis, does the location present a potential for serious complications (i.e., potential for hemorrhage or obstruction of blood flow due to the tumor located next to blood vessels)?

g) Is the wound malodorous or fungating?

h) A nutritional assessment is important, as malnutrition can impede proper wound healing and also cause pressure ulcer formation

2. Alteration in Oral Mucous Membranes

a) Patient history of mouth dryness or sore mouth

b) Review of medications which may cause oral membrane alterations (i.e., antibiotics, chemotherapy drugs such as IV 5-Fluouracil, anticholinergics)

c) Examination of internal and external oral mucosa:

(1) Dry, cracked lips

(2) Sores or white patches on buccal membranes, oropharynx or tongue

(3) Bleeding of gums, lips, or tongue

d) Patient's current oral hygiene regimen

e) Patient and family knowledge of etiology and management of altered oral mucous membranes

3. Pruritis

a) History of itching (including when, how long, what is tolerable)

b) Assessment of skin

(1) Presence of rashes or lesions

(2) Presence of abrasions from frequent scratching

(3) Overall skin integrity

c) Review plan of care for medications that may cause pruritis

D. Diagnoses

1. Impaired skin integrity, oral, related to dry mouth, oral lesions, infection

2. Impaired skin integrity related to immobility and pressure over bony prominences

3. Impaired skin integrity related to tumor necrosis or fistula

4. Pain related to altered skin or oral mucous membranes or pruritis

5. Body image disturbance related to malodorous or unsightly wounds

6. Patient/family knowledge deficit related to etiology and management of wounds, altered oral mucous membranes, or pruritis

E.   Planning and Intervention

1.   Wound management

a)   Relieve pressure

(1)   Turn at least every two hours

(2)   Place patient on pressure relief and pressure reduction support surfaces

b)   Reduce friction and shearing forces

(1)   Teach family proper techniques for moving patient in bed; physical therapy referral may be indicated

(2)   Use transparent dressings or elbow and knee protectors

c)   Consult team dietitian for nutritional assessment and plan of care

d)   Consult enterostomal therapy (ET) nurse for wound management plan, if appropriate

e)   Consult Agency for Healthcare Research and Quality (AHRQ) (formerly AHCPR) guidelines for skin and wound care

f)   Wounds should be cleansed and irrigated with normal saline prior to being dressed

(1)   Irrigation with low pressure (pouring directly from the bottle or using bulb or piston syringe) if wound has granulation tissue present and very little serous to serosanguineous exudate[2]

(2)   Irrigation with high pressure (35cc syringe with 19 gauge IV cannula attached) if wound has debris, eschar, or moderate to large amount of exudate (especially purulent)[2]

(3)   Dressing selection

(a)   The following should be considered when selecting a dressing[1]

(i)   Moist wound bed

(ii)   Dry surrounding skin

(iii)   Exudate control

(iv)   Caregiver time

(b)   If wounds are malodorous, special dressings are required to assist with odor control

(c)   Table I lists different types of dressings and the types of wounds for which they are appropriate

(4)   Assure adequate pain control prior to changing dressings; utilize topical pain relievers as appropriate for ongoing pain (i.e., topical xylocaine, cold packs)

2.   Alteration in oral mucous membranes

   a)   Xerostomia

      (1)   Stimulate salivation

         (a)   Peppermint water

         (b)   Gum, mints, hard candy (preferably sugar free to protect teeth)

         (c)   Ice chips or frequent sips of water

         (d)   Pilocarpine 2.5 mg po tid, titrate to 10 mg po tid; do not use in patients with severe COPD or bowel obstruction[3]

   b)   Utilize saliva substitutes

      (1)   Ice chips or frequent sips of water

      (2)   Artificial saliva

   c)   Treat dehydration

      (1)   Ice chips or frequent sips of water

      (2)   Offer fluids throughout the day, especially with meals

      (3)   Humidify the room

      (4)   Place spray bottle and moistened oral swabs close to patient (avoid lemon-glycerin swabs)

   d)   Review medications, and alter regimen if appropriate

3.   Sore mouth due to oral candida, herpetic lesions, mucositis or stomatitis

   a)   For candida, nystatin swish and swallow or fluconazole

   b)   Around-the-clock mouth care at least every two to four hours with moistened oral swabs and saline mouth rinse, if patient is able; be sure to apply water-soluble lubricant to lips

   c)   1:4 hydrogen peroxide and water rinse for mucous or hard debris in mouth[4]

   d)   Do not serve hot or overly spicy foods; serve softened and moist foods rather than dry

   e)   Several oral medications and medicated mouthwash cocktails are available for mouth pain and lesions. Some examples are:

      (1)   Topical morphine

      (2)   Viscous lidocaine

      (3)   Cocktail of Milk of Magnesia, diphenhydramine, and viscous lidocaine

      (4)   Sucralfate slurry

   f)   PCA with IV Morphine may be used for severe oropharyngeal pain[5]

4.   Pruritis Interventions

    a)   Non-pharmacologic measures

        (1)   Avoid skin irritants that may cause dryness or additional moisture[4]

            (a)   Alcohol

            (b)   Tight or heavy clothing

            (c)   Frequent bathing with harsh soaps and hot water

        (2)   Avoid heat, maintain cool room temperatures; keep the patient cool to avoid sweating, and frequently cleanse the skin with neutral pH cleansers and tepid water

        (3)   Cool starch baths

        (4)   Cold compresses can decrease itching; make sure to assess skin frequently during application, and do not apply if patient's peripheral vascular system is compromised

        (5)   Apply lubricating ointments or creams to skin (i.e., lanolin) to avoid excessive drying

        (6)   Avoid alcohol, foods/drinks containing caffeine, theophylline

    b)   Pharmacologic Measures

        (1)   Antihistamines such as hydroxyzine (Atarax®) and diphenhydramine (Benadryl®)

        (2)   Topical corticosteroids can be used for acute localized itching, but should be avoided for chronic pruritis[5]

        (3)   Ondansetron has been used in cholestatic, uremic, and opioid-induced pruritis[6]

        (4)   Antifungal creams for pruritis related to candida

        (5)   Transcutaneous electrical nerve stimulation (TENS) units may be helpful in localized pruritis[6, 4]

F.   Patient/Family Education

1.   Wounds

    a)   Demonstrate correct positioning to maximize pressure relief. Explain importance of changing patient's position every two hours, when appropriate, even if the patient is sitting in a chair

    b)   Demonstrate proper technique in moving patient up in bed to reduce friction and shearing force

    c)   Demonstrate correct procedures for cleansing and dressing wounds

    d)   Explain possible complications with tumor necrotic wounds; prepare family for bleeding or airway concerns and management

    e)   Explain management of ostomy bags if fistula present

2. Altered oral mucous membranes

    a) Demonstrate proper technique for oral care; explain importance of frequent oral care

    b) Explain medication usage and potential side effects

    c) Introduce non-pharmacologic methods for preventing and relieving dry and sore oral mucous membranes

3. Pruritis

    a) Explain etiology of pruritis

    b) Explain ways of preventing pruritis (keep skin clean and dry, avoid soaps, etc.)

    c) Explain actions of medications and potential side effects

    d) Introduce non-pharmacologic methods for preventing and relieving pruritis (See Section E, 4 a) above)

G. Evaluate

1. Wounds

    a) Response of patient/family to teaching

    b) Effectiveness of interventions (i.e., is wound healing?)

    c) Need for change in plan (i.e., change in dressing, referral to ET nurse)

    d) Patient/family understanding of treatment and prevention of further alteration of skin integrity

2. Altered oral mucous membranes and pruritis

    a) Response to interventions and patient/family teaching

    b) Effectiveness of interventions: are patient/family satisfied with outcome?

    c) Medication effects and side effects

    d) Patient/family understanding of treatment and prevention of further alteration

H. Revise plan according to findings from ongoing evaluations, changes in patient status or family needs

Table 1: Indications and Uses for Dressings

Type of Dressing	Indications and Uses
Semipermeable film	Protects very early damage from shear forces. Prevents bacterial contamination. Maintains humidity in shallow ulcers, producing ideal conditions for granulation and healing. Provides immediate pain relief. Best applied when there is no exudation from the wound.
Hydrocolloids	For low-exudate wounds. Maintains moist environment. Fluidizes to produce a gel useful for debridement. Provides environment for granulation. Available as a paste to fill wound cavities.
Alginates	For heavy exudates; controls secretion and bacterial contamination by absorption and formation of hydrophilic gel.
Hydrogels/xerogel	For debridement in the presence of slough and infection: rehydrates eschar and makes it easier to remove.
Enzymatic	For eschar and necrotic tissue; loosens necrotic tissue by liquefaction, thereby aiding in its removal (Protect edges of wound with zinc paste and apply to eschar under an occlusive dressing).
Polysaccharide dextranomer	For exudative, infected wounds; on contact with wound exudates the beads absorb fluid and swell, forming a gel; bacteria and dead cells are drawn away from the wound. Applied every 24 hours until wound is clean and granulation tissue is developing.
Charcoal	Malodorous infected pressure sores: adsorbs bacteria, cellular debris, toxins, and odors.

Reprinted with permission from: Waller, A., & Caroline, N. L. *Handbook of Palliative Care in Cancer,* 2nd ed. Boston: Butterworth-Heinemann, 2000: 97.

III. Altered Mental Status: Confusion, Delirium, Terminal Restlessness, Agitation

    A. Confusion/Delirium/Agitation

        1. Definitions:

            a) **Confusion**

                (1) Clouding of consciousness, memory impairment

                (2) Change in cognition/impaired cognitive function, impaired perceptions and emotional disturbances

                (3) May be accompanied by reduced level of consciousness, disorientation and misperceptions

            b) **Delirium**

                (1) Exaggerated emotions or memories with aggression, paranoia or terror displayed

                (2) Disturbance of consciousness with reduced ability to focus

                (3) Disturbance develops over a short period of time (hours or days) and tends to fluctuate over the course of the day

            c) **Agitation**

                (1) Can occur at any time during a disease process and is an objective result of confusion or delirium

                (2) A group of symptoms that may include physically and/or verbally aggressive behaviors, hiding or hoarding behaviors and physically nonaggressive behaviors, i.e., pacing, inappropriate dressing/undressing, repetitive actions[7]

        2. Potential Etiologies

            a) Medications: opioids, phenothiazines, benzodiazepines, anticholinergics, beta-blockers, diuretics, dopaminergics, steroids, atropine, phenytoin, H_2 antagonists, digoxin only when toxic

            b) Unrelieved pain, discomfort or other unrelieved symptoms

            c) Full bladder or bowel

            d) Infection (UTI, lung, septicemia)

            e) Brain tumor, primary or metastatic

            f) Cardiac or respiratory failure

            g) Metabolic disturbance (calcium, urea nitrogen, glucose, sodium)

            h) Nicotine, alcohol, drug withdrawal

            i) Extreme, uncontrolled anxiety

3.   Assess for:

    a)   Confusion vs. delirium using available tools such as those listed below[7]

        (1)   Memorial Delirium Assessment Scale (MDAS)

        (2)   Delirium Rating Scale (DRS)

        (3)   Neecham Confusion Scale (NCS)

        (4)   Confusion Assessment Method (CAM)

    b)   Differentiation between hyperalert-hyperactive and hypoalert-hypoactive variants of delirium

    c)   Patient's previous personality and emotional coping abilities

    d)   Alcohol, drug use history; recent nicotine, alcohol or drug use

    e)   Signs of infection

        (1)   Fever, flushing, tachycardia, tachypnea, perspiration

        (2)   These symptoms of infection may not be present in persons with immunosuppression due to corticosteroids, chemotherapy, disease process or in the elderly

    f)   Abdominal examination: palpate for bladder or bowel, abdominal distention

    g)   Bowel history, noting time and character of last bowel movement; rectal examination for impaction

    h)   If diabetic history or currently on corticosteroids, capillary blood glucose

    i)   Lab studies including: BUN, creatinine, electrolytes, glucose, calcium

    j)   Consider midstream clean-catch urinalysis, culture and sensitivity

    k)   Neurologic status: dysphasia, weakness, bilateral strength, coordination; poor coordination

    l)   Patient safety

    m)   Patient and family coping with change in mental status and ways of managing patient

4.   Potential diagnoses

    a)   Altered mental status changes potentially related to: (etiology)

    b)   High safety risk for fall related to altered mental status

    c)   Impaired bowel function related to constipation from (etiology)

    d)   Impaired bladder function related to retention from (etiology)

    e)   Disturbed physiologic response to infection related to corticosteroid use, aging

    f)   Impaired physiologic response related to alcohol, drugs, medication

    g)   Risk for alcohol, drug withdrawal due to recent use

5. Planning and Intervention

   a) Etiology of altered mental status will determine intervention plan

   b) Effective pain control and control of other disabling symptoms

   c) Assess patient's current medications for compliance, effects and iatrogenic effects (side effects) contributing to altered mental status

   d) Review with MD; consider discontinuation or reduction of medications thought to be contributing to patient's confusion

   e) Correct metabolic imbalance, if appropriate

   f) Support alcohol, drug withdrawal chemically as indicated

   g) Treat infection as appropriate

   h) For impaction, disimpact; establish aggressive bowel regimen

   i) For urine retention, straight or retention catheter to relieve

   j) Support withdrawal from nicotine, alcohol or drugs if withdrawal is contributing to agitation

   k) Reassure patient and family and provide constant, consistent reorientation of confused patient

   l) Provide for patient's safety; follow agency/institutional policy regarding the use of restraints, both chemical and physical

   m) Avoid sedation if possible

   n) Psychotropic drugs do not reverse confusion or altered mental status, but they may calm distressing agitation, paranoia or hallucinations

      (1) Haloperidol, chlorpromazine are first line

      (2) Risperidol is particularly helpful in managing agitation and hallucinations in the elderly

6. Patient and family education

   a) Since confusion is most distressing to patients and families, much education and support is required

   b) Intermittent nature of most confusion

   c) Expected therapeutic response to interventions

   d) Expected medication effects and potential side effects

   e) Safety needs of patient during periods of confusion, agitation

   f) Importance of compliance with bowel regimen, bladder emptying

7. Evaluate

   a) Effectiveness of interventions:

      (1) Medications

      (2) Non-pharmacologic interventions

      b)   Family participation and coping

      c)   Reassess to determine additional needs

8.   Revise plan according to findings from ongoing evaluations, changes in patient status or family needs

B. Terminal restlessness

1.   Definitions

      a)   Excessive restlessness, increased mental and physical activity[8]

      b)   Commonly seen features are frequent, non-purposeful motor activity, inability to concentrate or relax, disturbances in sleep or rest patterns, potential for progression to agitation[9]

2.   Potential etiologies include:

      a)   Full bladder, constipation/impaction

      b)   Hypoxia, dyspnea

      c)   Left ventricular failure, decreased cardiac output

      d)   Uncontrolled pain

      e)   Denial, anxiety, unfinished emotional, and/or spiritual issues

      f)   Also consider the possible etiologies listed above for confusion/delirium/agitation

3.   Assess for:

      a)   Etiology of terminal restlessness

      b)   Emotional, spiritual history related to issues, personal peace, resolution

      c)   Shortness of breath or labored breathing; lung sounds

      d)   Bladder and bowel status

      e)   Hallucinations, muscle twitching or jerking

      f)   "Sundowning"

4.   Potential diagnoses

      a)   Disturbed mental status related to: [etiology]

      b)   High risk for injury due to agitation and uncontrolled restlessness

      c)   Family coping impairment related to severe stress of uncontrolled agitation

5.   Plan and interventions

      a)   Etiology of restlessness will determine intervention plan

      b)   Disimpaction, bladder relief if distended

    c)   Consult MD for pharmacologic management. Medications may include:

        (1)   Opioid analgesics for pain and sedation

        (2)   Antipsychotics

            (a)   Chlorpromazine (Thorazine®)

            (b)   Haloperidol (Haldol®)

            (c)   Risperidone (Risperdal®) is particularly helpful in managing agitation and hallucinations in the elderly

        (3)   Barbiturates

            (a)   Phenobarbital (Luminal®)

            (b)   Pentobarbital (Nembutal®)

        (4)   Benzodiazepines

            (a)   Lorazepam (Ativan®) (if no delirium)

            (b)   Diazepam (Valium®)

            (c)   Midazolam (Versed®)

    d)   Medications should be given by the least invasive route possible: oral, rectal, transdermal, subcutaneous or intravenous; intramuscular route should be used only if absolutely necessary

    e)   Regular assessment of medication effects

    f)   Pharmacologic control of muscle twitching, jerking

    g)   Pastoral and psychological support of patient and family for emotional and spiritual issues

    h)   Non-pharmacologic approaches including:

        (1)   Subdued, quiet, calm environment

        (2)   Consistent, familiar faces and staff

        (3)   Calm and reassuring presence

        (4)   Relaxation techniques

            (a)   Visualization

            (b)   Distraction

            (c)   Massage

        (5)   Pet therapy, if appropriate

6.   Family education

    a)   Calm environment, presence with minimal stimulation

    b)   Non-pharmacologic methods for cueing patient with relaxation, visualization, massage, music, distraction

      c)   Expected therapeutic response to medications and potential side effects

      d)   Prepare family for patient's sedation response to medications

      e)   Prepare family for patient's death; encourage speaking with/to patient and using "letting go" language and phrases if family able

7. Evaluate

      a)   Effectiveness of interventions

         (1)   Medications

         (2)   Non-pharmacologic interventions

      b)   Family participation and coping

      c)   Reassess to determine additional needs

8. Revise plan according to findings from ongoing evaluations, changes in patient status or family needs

IV. Anorexia and Cachexia

A. Definitions

1. Anorexia: Loss of appetite or inability to take in nutrients

2. Cachexia: Weight loss and wasting due to inadequate intake of nutrients

B. Possible etiologies

1. Anorexia

      a)   Pain

      b)   Constipation

      c)   Nausea and vomiting

      d)   Alteration in oral mucous membranes (candidiasis, xerostomia, mucositis)

      e)   Impaired gastric emptying

      f)   Change of taste in foods (dysgeusia); change in smell of foods

      g)   Altered mental status (depression, dementia, confusion, anxiety)

      h)   Fatigue

      i)   Medications (opioids, antibiotics)

      j)   Radiation or chemotherapy

2. Cachexia

    a) Increased nutritional losses related to etiologies associated with anorexia

    b) Increased nutritional losses associated with[4]:

        (1) Bleeding

        (2) Diarrhea

        (3) Malabsorption of nutrients (i.e., pancreatic cancer)

    c) Metabolic Disorders

        (1) Abnormal protein metabolism (negative nitrogen balance and decreased muscle mass)

        (2) Abnormal carbohydrate metabolism due to inefficient energy metabolism

        (3) Abnormal lipid metabolism (overall depletion of total body fat)

        (4) Change in fluid and electrolyte balance (increase in extracellular fluid and total body sodium and decrease in intracellular fluid and total body potassium)[4]

C. Assess For:

1. History of loss of appetite, including reasons for loss (i.e., change in taste or smell, dysphagia, nausea and vomiting)

2. Patient food likes and dislikes

3. Oral mucosa for dryness, sores, candidiasis

4. Medications that may cause a decrease in appetite

5. Symptoms of malabsorption, such as diarrhea

6. Decrease in bowel sounds

7. Signs and symptoms of constipation or fecal impaction

8. Signs and symptoms of metabolic disorder, such as hypoglycemia, hypernatremia, hypokalemia, dehydration, hypercalcemia

9. Patient/family knowledge of etiology of anorexia and cachexia

D. Potential Diagnoses

1. Nutrition less than body requirements related to anorexia

2. Fatigue, related to decreased nutritional intake secondary to anorexia

3. Body image disturbance, related to cachexia

4. Anxiety related to inability to eat as desired

5. Patient/family knowledge deficit related to etiology and management of anorexia/cachexia

E. Plan/Interventions[4]

1. Encourage patient and family to prepare foods the patient likes and have those foods available whenever the patient requests them

2. Refer to Interdisciplinary Team dietitian

3. Give patient permission to eat less than before

4. Encourage small, frequent meals rather than three large meals

5. Avoid strong odors; allow food to cool before serving

6. Serve small portions with a pleasing appearance

7. In cases where anorexia is due to nausea/vomiting, altered oral mucous membranes, constipation, or diarrhea (See sections in this chapter on treating these symptoms.)

8. Encourage nutritional supplements

9. Enteral feedings may be appropriate in certain cases if patient's GI function is adequate for digestion/absorption

10. Parenteral nutrition support (total or peripheral parenteral nutrition, i.e., TPN or PPN) if indicated and desired by patient/family (rare in hospice setting)

11. Pharmacologic interventions (see Table 2)

F. Patient/Family Education

1. Encourage patient to eat as often as desired, but assure patient it is okay not to eat if it is uncomfortable.

2. Explain dying process to patient/family, especially that anorexia is normal in last days of life

3. Encourage open communication regarding nutrition

G. Evaluate

1. Has patient's appetite and nutritional intake increased, if this was a goal?

2. Patient/family response to interventions. Are they satisfied with outcome?

3. Are symptoms contributing to anorexia/cachexia treated, if appropriate?

H. Revise plan according to findings from ongoing evaluations, changes in patient status, or family needs

Table 2: Anorexia/Cachexia: Pharmacologic Interventions

Class of Drug	Example(s)	Comments
Gastrokinetic Agents	Metoclopramide 10 mg po tid	Useful in patients complaining of nausea or early satiety.
Corticosteroids	Dexamethasone 4 mg po q am, then taper gradually to the minimum effective dosage	Highly effective in improving appetite in the short term, with side effects at the dosage recommended; may lose efficacy after a few weeks.
Progesterone Analogs	Megestrol acetate 400–800 mg po qd Medroxy-progesterone acetate 100 mg po tid	80% of patients will show improvement in appetite; significant decreases in nausea and vomiting occur in more than 50%; abnormalities of taste are often reduced, and weight gain (of fat, fluid and lean body mass) is seen in nearly all patients except those in the most terminal stages. Treatment with recommended dosage costs $2/day (more expensive but has fewer side effects than steroids)
Cannabinoids	Dronabinol 2.5 mg po bid 1 hour pc	An effective appetite stimulant in low doses, without the usual side effects of drowsiness and muddled thinking
Alcohol	1 glass of beer or sherry before meals	May improve appetite and morale in patients who enjoyed a drink before dinner when they were well.
Vitamins	Multivitamins Vitamin C, 500 mg qid	Anecdotal evidence of improved appetite (may be due to placebo effect).

Reprinted with permission from Waller, A. and Caroline N. L. *Handbook of Palliative Care in Cancer*, 2nd ed. Boston: Butterworth-Heinemann, 2000: 152

V.   Ascites

A.   Definition: the accumulation of excessive fluid in the peritoneal cavity

B.   Possible etiologies

1.   Portal hypertension: Obstruction of portal vessels, causing leakage into abdominal cavity. Usually due to:

a)   Cirrhosis

b)   Cancer (ovarian, endometrial, breast, colon, pancreatic, gastric, lymphoma, liver)

c)   Cardiac dysfunction: congestive heart failure, constrictive pericarditis

2.   Decreased plasma oncotic pressure: Decrease in plasma albumin levels, causing fluid to leave plasma and accumulate in abdomen. Usually due to:

a)   Cirrhosis

b)   Nephrotic syndrome

c)   Malnutrition

3.   Lymphatic obstruction due to tumor infiltration in the abdomen, causing a buildup of fluid in the abdomen.

C.   Assess for:

1.   History relating to etiology (i.e., liver damage, cancer, alcoholism)

2.   Weight gain

3.   Tachycardia, dyspnea, orthopnea

4.   Decrease in mobility: unable to bend or sit straight

5.   Peripheral edema

6.   Abdominal signs:

a)   Measure abdominal girth every visit

b)   Fluid wave test

c)   Shifting dullness test

d)   Abdominal striae

e)   Distended abdominal wall veins

7.   Dehydration

8.   Anorexia/early satiety

D. **Diagnoses**

1. Pain, related to increasing abdominal girth

2. Immobility, and fatigue secondary to ascites

3. Impaired gas exchange related to ascites

4. Activity intolerance related to ascites

5. Patient/family knowledge deficit related to etiology and treatment of ascites

E. **Planning and Intervention**

1. Treatment is determined by the extent of fluid accumulation

2. Analgesics (usually low-dose opioids) can be used for the pain and discomfort of abdominal distention

3. Fluid and sodium restriction: limit fluid to 500–1000 cc/day, and sodium to 200–1000 mg/day; may not be successful in malignant ascites[10]

4. Diuretics may be added if fluid and sodium restriction has not been successful after four to five days; spironolactone is drug of choice, with furosemide added if spironolactone alone is not successful

5. Paracentesis may be indicated for palliation if the patient's comfort is extremely compromised

6. Palliative chemotherapy may reduce tumor size and invasion, which may be causing ascites

7. Close monitoring of intake and output may be needed, depending on where patient is on disease trajectory

F. **Patient/Family Education**

1. Discuss dietary measures (fluid and sodium restriction) to reduce ascites

2. Explain effects of medication and potential side effects (including dehydration for diuretics)

3. Explain skin problems associated with ascites, and demonstrate proper measures for maintaining skin integrity

4. Discuss signs and symptoms of infection if paracentesis is part of the treatment plan

G. **Evaluate**

1. Effectiveness of interventions and patient/family teaching (are patient/family satisfied with outcome?)

2. Medication effectiveness and presence of side effects

3. Skin integrity

H. **Revise Plan according to findings from ongoing evaluations, changes in patient status or family needs**

VI. Aphasia

A. Definition: absence or impairment of ability to communicate through speech, writing or signs

B. Possible etiologies

1. Left cerebral hemisphere lesion from infarct, hemorrhage, tumor, trauma or degeneration

2. Advanced dementia, cerebral vascular disease

C. Assess for:

1. Types of aphasia

   a) Sensory (receptive) aphasia: inability to comprehend spoken or written words

   b) Motor (expressive) aphasia: comprehension but inability or impairment of speech

   c) Global (sensory & motor) aphasia: failure of all forms of communication

2. Impairment of patient's ability to communicate pain, comfort needs

3. Difficulty in assessment of patient orientation, knowledge, judgment, abstraction, calculation ability and emotional responses, which can impact patient education, safety management

4. Caregiver's abilities, willingness to interpret patient's needs

5. Patient and family frustration, anxiety about deficits in communication

D. Potential Diagnoses

1. Speech and communication impairment related to type of aphasia and probable etiology

2. Compromised patient, family coping, stress, tolerance related to onset of aphasia

3. Patient knowledge deficit related to adjustment to impairment, disease process, therapeutic regimen related to aphasia

E. Planning and Intervention

1. Model acceptance and patience in communication

2. Speech therapy clinician consultation for recommendations for improving communication

3. Writing or picture boards for expressive aphasia

4. Ongoing inquiry and monitoring of patient's non-verbal behaviors for anxiety, pain, discomfort

5. Consistency in communication with patient from family and interdisciplinary team members

F.   Patient/family education

1.   Instruct, support caregiver/family in learning patient's non-verbal cues and developing signs, signals for communicating patient's needs: e.g. pain relief, toileting, thirst, hunger, repositioning, emotional feelings

2.   Instruct in reducing excessive stimuli in environment that can distract communication

G.   Evaluate for effectiveness of interventions, specifically

1.   Development of alternate communication tools

2.   Patient, family coping and adaptation

3.   Patient comfort: symptom progression or relief (pain or other)

4.   Patient needs being met

5.   Interdisciplinary team consistency

H.   Revise Plan according to findings from ongoing evaluations, changes in patient status or family needs

VII. Bladder Spasms

A.   Definition: intermittent, painful contractions of the detrusor muscle, leading to suprapubic pain and urgency

B.   Possible etiologies

1.   Indwelling catheter and/or problems associated with indwelling catheters (obstruction, size or balloon too large)

2.   Urinary tract infection

3.   Encroachment on bladder or urethra by tumor or impacted feces

4.   Radiation or chemotherapy cystitis

5.   Urethral obstruction by tumors or blood clots

6.   Neurologic disorders: stroke, spinal cord lesions, multiple sclerosis

C.   Assess for:

1.   Possible etiologies as documented in the medical history (history of bladder or prostate cancer, neurologic disorders, recent radiation or chemotherapy)

2.   Signs and symptoms of urinary tract infection

3.   Indwelling catheter function, assess catheter and balloon size as possible source of spasm

4.   Hematuria

5.   Food and fluid intake: Some foods aggravate symptoms; adequate fluid intake important for urinary tract health

6.   Presence of fecal impaction

D.   Potential Diagnoses

1.   Pain related to bladder spasm secondary to obstruction/infection/disease process

2.   Altered urinary elimination related to bladder spasm

3.   Patient and family knowledge deficit related to disease process, management of indwelling catheter, and treatment of bladder spasm

E.   Planning and Intervention: etiology will guide treatment

1.   Presence of indwelling catheter

a)   Reassess the need for Foley catheter

b)   Change catheter to appropriate size

c)   Partially deflate balloon

d)   Gently irrigate with normal saline

e)   May need to initiate continuous saline irrigation if etiology is related to blood clots

2.   Urinary tract infection

a)   Antibiotics

b)   Reassess the need for Foley catheter

c)   Change catheter if catheterized

d)   Increase oral fluid intake if feasible

3.   Disimpact if etiology is fecal impaction

4.   Non-pharmacologic measures: Assisting the patient to void every 4 hours, sitting or standing to void, teach relaxation techniques

5.   Pharmacologic measures: Antispasmodic drugs such as oxybutynin (Ditropan®); NSAIDs; Belladonna and Opium (B & O) suppositories

F.   Patient/Family Education

1.   Explain etiology of bladder spasm and measures to reduce symptoms

2.   Demonstrate proper catheter care and explain signs and symptoms of catheter obstruction

3.   Explain signs and symptoms of urinary tract infection

4.   Teach expected medication effects and potential side effects

G.   Evaluate

1.   Effectiveness of interventions and/or medications in decreasing pain related to bladder spasm

2.   Effectiveness of antibiotic therapy, if appropriate

3.   Patient/family understanding of interventions and medication regimen and recognition of symptoms

H.   **Revise Plan according to findings from ongoing evaluations, changes in patient status or family needs**

VIII.   Bowel Incontinence

A.   **Definition: the inability to control bowel movements.**

B.   **Possible etiologies**

1.   Obstruction, including fecal impaction or tumor (overflow incontinence)

2.   Diarrhea (See Section XI: Diarrhea)

3.   Sphincter damage due to rectal carcinoma, recto-vaginal fistula, or inflammatory bowel disease involving the rectum

4.   Sensory or motor dysfunction of the rectosphincter due to spinal cord lesions or compression, multiple sclerosis, diabetes

5.   Changes in sphincter tone related to age or spinal cord compression

6.   Dementia or mobility related (unable to verbalize or recognize need or unable to reach the toilet)

C.   **Assess for:**

1.   Rectal urgency and passage of loose or formed stool without patient control; incontinence of formed stool usually related to dementia[11], fecal impaction

2.   Functional status: is patient able to reach toilet?

3.   Neurologic and sensory function

4.   Skin integrity

D.   **Potential diagnoses**

1.   Bowel incontinence related to obstruction, diarrhea, neurosensory dysfunction, or impaired cognition

2.   Risk for impaired skin integrity related to bowel incontinence

3.   Patient/family knowledge deficit related to etiology and management of bowel incontinence

4.   Patient/family anxiety related to bowel incontinence

E.   **Planning and Intervention: Etiology will guide interventions**

1.   Review bowel regimen and adjust laxative dose as needed if patient is taking opioids for pain

2.   Utilize opioids for constipating effect (codeine most effective)

3.   Disimpact if fecal impaction is causing incontinence; may need opioid or anxiolytic prior to disimpaction

4. Modify dietary practices if appropriate and as tolerated

   a) Decrease fiber intake to reduce bulk formation of stool

   b) Increase fluid intake of lukewarm, room temperature, or cool beverages (very cold or hot liquids can act as stimulants)

   c) Avoid spicy, greasy, rich, and fried foods; avoid caffeine and high amounts of milk products

   d) Incorporate bananas, rice, applesauce into diet; eat several small frequent meals rather than large meals

5. Alter environment to place patient closer to toileting facilities

6. Initiate a bowel routine (i.e., taking patient to toilet after eating)

7. Maintain skin integrity with adequate skin cleansing and liberal use of skin protectant ointment

8. Utilize incontinence products

F. Patient/Family Education

1. Explain etiology of bowel incontinence, and appropriate interventions relative to the etiology

2. Explain effects of medication and potential side effects

3. Demonstrate correct hygiene and skin care techniques to prevent skin breakdown

4. Explain safety measures if altering environment for ease in toileting (i.e., have patient call for assistance, bowel routine, assuring clear path to bathroom)

G. Evaluate

1. Effectiveness of interventions and patient/family teaching (Are patient/family satisfied with outcome?)

2. Medication effectiveness and presence of side effects.

3. Skin integrity

4. Patient safety

H. Revise plan according to findings from ongoing evaluations, changes in patient status or family needs

IX. Bowel Obstruction

A. Definition: occlusion of the lumen of the intestine, delaying or preventing the normal passage of feces

B. Possible etiologies

1. External compression of the lumen (i.e., tumor enlargement, metastases, adhesions, organomegaly)

2. Internal occlusion of the lumen (i.e., tumor, intussusception)

3. Ischemic or inflammatory processes (i.e., Crohn's disease, diverticulitis, peritonitis, pancreatitis, hernia)

4. Fecal blockage (severe constipation can mimic obstruction)

5. Adynamic ileus (i.e., pneumonia, metabolic/electrolyte problems)

6. Metabolic disorders (i.e., Crohn's disease, hypokalemia)

7. Drugs (i.e., diuretics can cause hypokalemia, which decreases peristalsis; opioids; chemotherapy)

8. Often more than one etiology is present when a bowel obstruction develops

C. Assess for:

1. History: predisposition to obstruction (cancer, pancreatitis, etc.), history of bowel habits, medication usage, history of pain

2. Pain

   a) Crampy, colicky pain in the middle to upper abdomen relieved with vomiting suggests a small bowel obstruction

   b) Crampy pain in the lower abdomen that increases over time suggests a large bowel obstruction

   c) Severe, steady pain is a sign of bowel strangulation

3. Abdominal Distention: present and possibly severe in obstruction of the large intestine; visible peristalsis may be present; patient may complain of constipation and bloating

4. Nausea and Vomiting: moderate to severe in small bowel obstruction, and can relieve pain. May develop later in obstruction of the large intestine

5. Bowel sounds: hyperactive sounds and borborygmi; hypoactive or absent sounds with adynamic ileus

6. Constipation and inability to pass flatus seen in complete obstruction

7. Diarrhea due to overflow of feces related to fecal impaction

8. Fever and chills could indicate bowel ischemia or strangulation

D. Possible Diagnoses

1. Pain related to bowel obstruction

2. Potential for fluid and electrolyte imbalances related to vomiting secondary to bowel obstruction

3. Anxiety related to pain and inability to defecate secondary to bowel obstruction

4. Nausea and vomiting related to bowel obstruction

5. Patient/family knowledge deficit related to etiology and treatment of bowel obstruction

E. Planning and Intervention

1. Disimpact if necessary, utilizing an opioid or anxiolytic if needed for patient comfort

2. Surgery may be considered if:

   a) This is patient's first obstruction

   b) The obstruction occurs in only one site

   c) The patient has a >2 months prognosis and good overall function[12]

   d) Surgery is not usually indicated for non-mechanical obstructions

3. Medication for pain including antispasmodics (loperamide or scopolomine), and opioids

4. Stimulant laxatives (senna, bisacodyl) and prokinetics (metoclopramide) should be discontinued if patient is experiencing colicky pain[11]

5. Medication for nausea and vomiting (if symptoms are distressful for patient) including promethazine, prochlorperazine, or haloperidol

6. Gastric decompression using NG suction may be necessary for relief of gastric distention and nausea; if symptoms persist, percutaneous gastrostomy placement can aid in venting

7. Oral fluids should be increased if tolerable and nausea and vomiting can be controlled; parenteral fluids may be considered if vomiting is not controlled and patient at risk for severe dehydration

8. Treat diarrhea or constipation according to interventions outlined in sections X and XI

F. Patient/family education

1. Explain etiology and treatment course of bowel obstruction

2. Explain medication effects and possible side effects

3. Demonstrate post-operative care of incisions/gastrostomy tube, if appropriate

4. Explain importance of bowel regime, and assist in initiating regime, if appropriate

G. **Evaluate**

1. Effectiveness of interventions and patient/family teaching

2. Effects and side effects of medications

3. Patient/family understanding of treatment and prevention of further obstruction

H. **Revise plan according to findings from ongoing evaluations, changes in patient status or family needs**

X. **Constipation**

A. **Definition: difficulty in passing stools or an incomplete or infrequent passage of hard stools**

B. **Possible etiologies**

1. Intestinal obstruction: tumors in bowel wall, external compression of the bowel by pelvic or abdominal tumors

2. Medications: Opioids, tricyclic antidepressants, phenothiazines, antacids, diuretics, iron, vincristine, anti-hypertensives, anticonvulsants, anticholinergics or drugs with anticholinergic effects, NSAIDs

3. Metabolic disorders: Hypercalcemia, hypokalemia, hypothyroidism

4. Other disease processes or disorders: colitis, diverticular disease

5. Dietary problems: Low fiber intake, inadequate fluid intake, dehydration

6. Neurologic: Confusion, depression, sedation

7. Weakness, inactivity, and immobility

8. Pain associated with constipation, including anal fissures or hemorrhoids, straining at stool, etc.

9. Decrease in privacy or unfamiliar toilet facilities; patient reluctant to ask for help in toileting (embarrassment, loss of independence, do not want to be a burden, etc.)

C. **Assess for:**

1. Bowel history

a) Last bowel movement and bowel movement prior to last

b) Amount, color, consistency

c) Straining or pain during defecation

d) Current bowel regimen: does patient need aids in defecation, such as laxatives, suppositories, or digital removal

2. Food and fluid intake

3. Mobility potential

4. Abdominal assessment: Abdominal distension and/or tenderness; may report feeling of fullness or bloating; bowel sounds may be normal or hypoactive; percussion reveals dullness in otherwise tympanic areas; may be able to palpate stool in colon

5. Increase in flatus

6. Nausea, vomiting

7. Rectal examination: Presence of hemorrhoids, anal fissures; digital examination might reveal hard stool or large amount of soft stool in rectum

8. Patient, family understanding of underlying cause of constipation, expected effects of medication or non-pharmacological remedies

D. Potential Diagnoses

1. Risk for constipation related to opioid or other constipating medication usage, immobility, decrease in food, fluid intake

2. Constipation related to opioid medication usage, immobility, decrease in food, fluid intake

3. Alteration in comfort related to constipation

4. Patient, family knowledge deficit related to appropriate bowel regimen

E. Planning and Intervention

1. Goal in control of opioid-induced constipation is prevention of constipation

2. Bowel obstruction should be ruled out and disimpaction considered if appropriate

    a) If digitally disimpacting, give an opioid or anxiolytic prior to intervention

    b) Digital disimpaction contraindicated in neutropenic or thrombocytopenic patients; may be contraindicated in end stage cardiac patients

3. Non-pharmacologic therapies

    a) Increase fluid intake: Water and fruit juices are most effective (prune juice is especially helpful)

    b) Encourage high-fiber foods; examples include: whole grain breads and cereals, bran cereal, fresh, canned, frozen or dried fruits and vegetables

    c) Increase activity, including active or passive range of motion if possible

    d) Ask patient what has been effective in the past

4. Pharmacologic therapies

    a) If patient is at risk for constipation, prophylactic stool softener and stimulant laxatives should be started (example: Peri-colace or senna with docusate sodium)[11]

    b) Patient may use own regimen, but regular use should be stressed, especially if using opioids

    c) If no bowel movement in three days, regardless of intake, fluids should be increased and an osmotic laxative (i.e., lactulose, sorbitol) started

    d) For continuing constipation, a glycerin or bisacodyl suppository or sodium biphosphate enema may be added[11]

    e) Discontinue medications that may cause constipation if not medically necessary (i.e., iron or calcium supplements)

5.   Rectal pain or discomfort: Consider hemorrhoid preparations or warm sitz baths (R/O herpes in the case of a patient with HIV disease)

F.   Patient/Family Education

1.   Explain etiology of constipation and instruct in ways to manage

a)   Non-pharmacological interventions: increased food/fluid intake, increase activity

b)   Pharmacological interventions

2.   Continually reinforce necessity of bowel regime, even if patient is not constipated

3.   Explain medication effects and possible side effects

4.   Reinforce that bowel movement should occur at least every three days, and further action should be taken if no bowel movement after this time

G.   Evaluate

1.   Effectiveness of bowel regime:

a)   How often is patient having bowel movement?

b)   Is patient having difficulty during passage of stool?

2.   Assess abdomen and rectum (externally and digitally, if appropriate)

3.   Patient, family understanding of bowel regime, including medications and non-pharmacologic measures to prevent constipation

H.   Revise plan according to findings from ongoing evaluations, changes in patient status, or family needs

XI.   Diarrhea

A.   Definition: the frequent passage of loose, unformed, liquid stool

B.   Possible etiologies

1.   Laxative therapy overuse or imbalance

2.   Side effect of other drugs (i.e., NSAIDs, antibiotics)

3.   Radiation and chemotherapy

4.   Food intolerances or tube feedings

5.   Malnutrition (cachexia related to cancer or AIDS)

6.   Surgical procedures: gastrectomy, ileal resection, colectomy

7.   Fecal impaction

8.   Infection (especially as seen in immunocompromised patients, such as those with AIDS and post-chemotherapy)

9.   Partial intestinal obstruction

10. Tumors: gastrointestinal and carcinoid tumors, pancreatic islet cell tumors, small cell lung tumors

11. Gastrointestinal disorders: inflammatory bowel disease, pancreatic insufficiency, diverticulitis, ulcerative colitis, Crohn's disease

12. Other chronic disorders such as diabetes and hyperthyroidism

C. Assess for:

1. History, including characteristic of stool, how often stool is occurring, medication usage, recent radiation or chemotherapy treatments or gastrointestinal surgery

2. Physical exam:

   a) Abdominal assessment: bowel sounds may be hyperactive (or hypoactive to absent if intestinal obstruction is present), patient reports of cramping or pain, palpable masses in abdomen may indicate partial obstruction

   b) Nature and consistency of stool (if available to assess): pancreatic insufficiency is indicated by steatorrhea (loose, pale, foul-smelling, greasy stool); fecal impaction may be indicated by small amounts of loose stool

3. Signs of dehydration

4. Skin integrity

D. Potential diagnoses

1. Diarrhea related to infection, metabolic disorders, medications or therapies, partial obstruction, malnutrition, or GI intolerance to food/feedings

2. Risk for impaired skin integrity related to diarrhea

3. Potential for fluid and electrolyte imbalance related to diarrhea

4. Patient/family knowledge deficit related to etiology and treatment of diarrhea

E. Planning and Intervention: Etiology will guide treatment options

1. Increase fluid intake, preferably with electrolyte replacement drinks

2. Clear liquid diet for first 24 hours, with light carbohydrates (rice, crackers, etc.), then advance as tolerated to diet high in protein and calories; avoid spicy, greasy, high-fiber foods and foods high in lactose or caffeine; small, frequent meals are usually better tolerated. Incorporate bananas, rice, applesauce into diet to help keep stool firm in consistency

3. Disimpact if necessary, utilizing opioids or anxiolytics prior to intervention, if needed for patient comfort

4. Discontinue laxatives if certain etiology of diarrhea is not due to impaction

5. Antidiarrheals: loperamide; diphenoxylate HCl with atropine (Absorbent and adsorbent agents do not work as fast, so are not indicated in advanced disease); opioids can also be considered if patient is not already taking

6. Pancreatic insufficiency: pancreatic enzymes with meals, with loperamide (slows peristalsis)

7.   Maintain skin integrity with adequate skin cleansing and liberal use of skin protectant ointment

F.   Patient/Family Education

1.   Explain etiology of diarrhea, and appropriate interventions relative to the etiology

2.   Explain effects of medication and potential side effects

3.   Demonstrate correct hygiene and skin care techniques to prevent skin breakdown

4.   Explain signs, symptoms, and treatment of dehydration

G.   Evaluate

1.   Effectiveness of interventions and patient/family teaching (Are patient/family satisfied with outcome?)

2.   Medication effectiveness and presence of side effects

3.   Skin integrity

4.   Fluid volume status

H.   Revise plan according to findings from ongoing evaluations, changes in patient status or family needs

XII.   Dysphagia/Odynophagia

A.   Dysphagia: a subjective awareness of difficulty in swallowing

1.   Possible etiologies

a)   Obstructive: cancer of esophagus and other cancers of the head and neck area, benign peptic stricture & lower esophageal ring (history of GERD [Gastroesophageal Reflux Disease]), compression of vessels or mediastinal nodes. This type of dysphagia is intermittent, usually occurring when eating or drinking; meat and bread are most difficult foods to swallow; some patients can tolerate only liquids[13]

b)   Motor: neuromuscular, esophageal dysfunction (stasis) related to smooth muscle hypertonia or dystonia: e.g. cardiospasm, esophageal aperistalsis, diffuse esophageal spasm (GERD), amyotrophic lateral sclerosis, scleroderma; this type of dysphagia is often for both solids and liquids[13]

B.   Odynophagia: is a report of painful swallowing

1.   Possible etiologies

a)   Inflammatory process: candidiasis, conditions favoring overgrowth of fungal *Candida albicans* e.g. broad spectrum antibiotics, diabetes mellitus, compromised cellular immunity (AIDS, leukemia, chemotherapy)

b)   Dry mucous membranes due to xerostomia (decreased quantity or quality of saliva) from radiotherapy, anticholinergic or other medications

c)   Corrosive esophagitis (ingestion of substance damaging to mucosa)

      d)   Broncho-esophageal fistula with chief complaint: "coughing after ingesting fluids"

C.   Assess for:

1. Etiology of dysphagia or odynophagia, which will direct intervention plan

2. If odynophagia only, treatment of underlying cause may relieve symptom:

    a)   Assess oral cavity including tongue, gingiva, mucosa, lips, presence and amount of saliva

    b)   Note onset and duration of painful swallowing

    c)   Assess voice quality, swallowing ability, oral hygiene

    d)   Oral intake: review 24 hour quantity food/liquid.

    e)   Review history for AIDS, diabetes, chemotherapy, radiotherapy

    f)   Review current medications for contributing agents (steroid inhalers, steroids, antibiotics, sulfa)

    g)   Presence of creamy white curd-like patches in oropharynx, tongue; patches usually scrape off easily with 4X4 gauze; may cause bleeding

3. Current nutritional status related to disease process, goals of therapies, patient and family expectations

4. If dysphagia, odynophagia are accompanied by anorexia, evaluate patient for disease progression, current nutritional status; discuss management options with interdisciplinary team, patient and family

D.   Potential Diagnoses

1. Swallowing impairment, nutritional impairment related to dysphagia X time or odynophagia X time

2. Oral mucous membranes impairment related to: candidiasis, mucositis, xerostomia

3. Patient, family knowledge deficit of: nutrition; types of food, liquids; safety in food selection, expected medication, therapy effects and side effects

E.   Planning and Intervention

1. If candidiasis: antifungal swish and swallow QID X 7–10 days; OR antifungal PO X 5–7days

2. If mucositis or esophagitis from radiotherapy: topical anesthetic, antihistamine, antacid combination e.g. lidocaine/diphenhydramine/antacid in 1:1:1 ratio as swish and swallow IF patient has gag reflex

3. If obstruction from tumors/nodes: limited dose steroids may reduce inflammatory edema

4. If neuro-motor etiology: speech therapy consult may be helpful to evaluate swallow and make recommendation

5. If dry mucosa induced from medications or radiotherapy: artificial saliva, lip balm, exquisite oral care, increase hydration

6. Determine food consistency best tolerated by patient: liquids may have thickening agents added to facilitate swallowing

7. If medications are etiology of dysphagia or odynophagia, consider alternative medicines if appropriate

8. Artificial feeding may be considered for obstructive or fistula processes in some palliative care situations depending upon the patient's place on the disease trajectory, current nutritional and functional status and other factors

F. Patient/family education

1. Importance of excellent oral hygiene

2. Avoid nicotine, alcohol and caffeine, which increase esophageal and vasospasm and have mucosal drying effects

3. Cool, non-irritating foods and liquids generally better tolerated

4. Encourage patient to chew food well and to avoid large boluses of meat, bread; modify food consistency if necessary, e.g., ground or pureed meats

5. Anticipated medication effects and potential side effects

G. Evaluate for effectiveness of interventions, specifically

1. Resolution of candidiasis

2. Improvement in mucosal lubrication

3. Oral hygiene

4. Nutritional status

5. Patient/family understanding of instructions, recommendations

H. Revise plan according to findings from ongoing evaluations, changes in patient status or family needs

XIII. Dyspnea/Cough

A. Definitions

1. Dyspnea: subjective sensation of shortness of breath

2. Cough: a natural defense of the body to prevent entry of foreign material into the respiratory tract[14]

B. Possible etiologies

1. Dyspnea: lung tumor or metastases, pleural effusion, COPD, CHF, ascites, pneumothorax, pulmonary embolism, anemia, neurologic insult

2. Cough: infection, inflammation, cardiac (left ventricular failure), pulmonary disease (pleural effusion, bronchospasm, bronchogenic cancer), medications (ACE inhibitors), smoke, tobacco abuse or irritation from second-hand smoke, allergic conditions, GERD

C.   **Assess for:**

1.   Dyspnea: etiology will direct intervention plan

a)   Onset of dyspnea. Respiratory rate, depth, quality of respiration, lung sounds, accessory muscle use, stridor

b)   Past interventions that have provided relief/comfort

c)   Appropriate use and understanding of current medications for relief of dyspnea and accompanying anxiety

d)   Whether patient is a carbon dioxide (CO_2) retainer; this will influence decisions regarding oxygen delivery rate, opioid and anxiolytic dosing

e)   Patient/family anxiety, coping, understanding of dyspnea triggers and etiology, and interventions to control dyspnea

2.   Cough: etiology will direct intervention plan

a)   History and physical to determine etiology and appropriate treatment

(4)   Productive vs. nonproductive cough

(5)   If productive, sputum quantity and appearance

(6)   Diagnostic studies as appropriate

b)   Effect of cough on patient/family's quality of life

c)   Need for cough suppressant OR cough expectorant based on etiology and patient need

D.   **Potential Diagnoses**

1.   Respiratory alteration related to: impairment of airway clearance, breathing pattern, or gas exchange

2.   Patient/family knowledge deficit of: etiology or triggers of dyspnea and/or cough, steps to relieve dyspnea or anxiety; medication use, effects or side effects

3.   Patient discomfort related to inability to control cough and/or mobilize secretions

4.   Patient/family anxiety related to perceived situational powerlessness, fear, breathing impairment

E.   **Planning and Intervention**[14]

1.   Review of medical history, progression of disease, current medications; etiology of dyspnea will direct intervention plan

2.   Nonpharmacologic interventions:

a)   Dyspnea:

(1)   Position patient in high Fowler's position as appropriate; COPD patients do better leaning forward with upper arms supported on a table

(2)   Encourage pursed lip breathing in COPD patients

(3)   Palliative thoracentesis or paracentesis may be considered in selected patients

        (4)   Model calm reassurance

        (5)   Encourage intake of nutrient-dense beverages (e.g., commercial supplements) if p.o. intake is limited because of dyspnea; liquids take less eating effort

        (6)   Fan directly in front of patient; cool room environment

        (7)   Complementary therapies such as relaxation techniques, guided imagery, therapeutic touch

        (8)   Oxygen as appropriate

    b)   Productive cough: chest physiotherapy (if able to tolerate), oxygen, humidity and suctioning, elevate head of bed, frequent sips of water, throat lozenges

3.   Pharmacologic interventions

    a)   Dyspnea and productive cough

        (1)   Opioids (PO, SL, SQ, IV or nebulized) for bronchodilation

            (a)   Start low and titrate dose slowly for opioid-naïve patients and patients with CO_2 retention

            (b)   Monitor respiratory rate and depth

        (2)   High dose steroids for obstructive or inflammatory etiologies

        (3)   Antibiotics for infection if appropriate

        (4)   Anxiolytic medications may help to reduce the anxiety that often accompanies dyspnea: use and titrate slowly in elderly and patients with CO_2 retention; monitor respiratory rate and depth

        (5)   For uncontrolled dyspnea in hospice home-care setting, may consider short-term inpatient management

        (6)   Sedation at end of life for refractory dyspnea is an option

    b)   Nonproductive cough: nonopioid (dextromethorphan (Robitussin®), benzonatate (Tessalon®)) or opioid antitussives, inhaled anesthetic (lidocaine, bupivacaine (Marcain®))

        (1)   Nebulized lidocaine 2% for 10 minutes q 2–6 hours

        (2)   NPO for 1 hour post treatment due to risk of aspiration from loss of gag reflex from anesthetic agent

F.   Patient/family education

1.   Reassurance and empowerment of patient/family by review, rehearsal of steps to take when patient's shortness of breath begins

2.   Treatment options, medication effects, side effects

3.   Demonstrate relaxation techniques when patient/family is not in crisis

4.   Instruct others not to crowd dyspneic person and to remain calm, in control of emotions

5.   Consistency in information with rehearsal, review by all members of the interdisciplinary team

G. **Evaluate**

    1. Understanding, compliance and effectiveness of medications for dyspneic episodes

    2. For patient, family coping; reduction of, improvement in management and control of dyspneic episodes

    3. For progression of disease process related to uncontrolled dyspnea

H. **Revise plan according to findings from ongoing evaluations, changes in patient status or family needs**

XIV. **Edema**

A. **Definition: presence of excessive fluid in the intercellular tissues especially in the subcutaneous tissues**

B. **Possible etiologies**

    1. Protein deficiency

    2. Obstruction of venous return: peritoneal tumors, DVT, CHF, superior vena cava syndrome (SVCS)

    3. Renal failure

    4. Lymphedema: blockage of lymphatic return in the periphery or the abdomen from surgical procedures, pressure from tumor

    5. Ascites of liver failure; peritoneal inflammation

C. **Assess for:**

    1. Review of medical history and progression of disease process

    2. Etiology of edema, which will direct intervention plan.

    3. New, increased or returning edema

    4. Extremity edema, pitting, non-pitting, tissue perfusion, warmth, cold, presence or absence of leaking from tissues.

    5. Superior Vena Cava Syndrome (SVCS):

        a) Upper body edema, i.e., papilledema, facial edema, distended neck veins, one or both arms depending on where the obstruction is located: note onset, tissues involved

        b) Other symptoms: dyspnea (most common), headache, chest pain, dry cough, visual or mental status changes, dizziness, vertigo

        c) SVCS is considered an oncologic emergency and may be palliated with radiotherapy with or without steroids depending on the etiology

        d) Not responsive to diuretics

    6. Ascites: abdomen size, tenderness, distention, fluid wave; if elevated diaphragm, may have dyspnea, pleural effusion

    7. Patient, family understanding of disease process related to poor perfusion, expected medication effects and possible side effects

D. Potential Diagnoses

1. Tissue perfusion alteration related to: peripheral edema, ascites, upper body, head and neck edema

2. Skin integrity impairment and risk related to poor perfusion, subcutaneous tissue edema, increased pressure points

3. Respiratory alteration related to gas exchange impairment (for dyspnea related to ascites, SVC syndrome)

4. Patient, family knowledge deficit of disease process, expected medication effects or possible side effects, non-pharmacologic measures

E. Planning and Intervention

1. Etiology of edema will direct intervention plan

2. Symptomatic relief of ascites: spironolactone (Aldactone®), paracentesis; diuretics are rarely successful in reducing ascites

3. Symptomatic relief of peripheral edema: compression stockings; diuretics usually appropriate when there are also crackles heard in lungs; meticulous skin care; active or passive exercise to help venous return if patient can tolerate; limb elevation above level of heart

4. Lymphedema

    a) Does not respond to diuretics unless there is a true peripheral edema component

    b) May not resolve despite elevation, compression stockings

    c) In the palliative care patient not actively dying, manual lymph drainage therapies may promote better quality of life

F. Patient/family education

1. Explain etiology of edema and instruct in ways to manage or reduce

2. Expected medication effects and possible side effects

3. Application of compression stockings prior to ambulation

4. Post paracentesis care

G. Evaluate

1. Effectiveness of medication

2. For level, return, extension of edema

3. Patient, family understanding of disease process, medications, application and use of compression stockings and/or manual lymph drainage therapies; non-pharmacologic interventions

H. Revise plan according to findings from ongoing evaluations, changes in patient status or family needs

XV. Extrapyramidal Symptoms (EPS)

    A.   Definition: involuntary movements, hyperkinetic (akathisia) or hypokinetic (dystonia); tardive dyskinesia is a late-effect, which may not respond to reversal therapies

    B.   Possible etiologies

        1.   Iatrogenic drug-induced from:

            a)   Neuroleptics

            b)   Phenothiazines: e.g. chlorpromazine (Thorazine®)

            c)   Butyrophenones: e.g. haloperidol (Haldol®)

            d)   Clozapine (Clozaril®)

            e)   Metoclopramide (Reglan®)

            f)   Opioids (myoclonus)

            g)   Others

        2.   Parkinson's disease, chorea

        3.   Cerebral lesions

    C.   Assess for:

        1.   Etiology of EPS from medical history, medication review which will direct intervention plan

        2.   Possible iatrogenic response to a medical therapy used to treat a symptom

        3.   Patient safety with ambulation, activities of daily living (ADL's)

        4.   Patient/family anxiety relating to EPS, understanding of medication effects and side effects

    D.   Diagnosis

        1.   Impaired physical mobility related to neurologic impairment caused by: etiology

        2.   Self-care deficit related to: immobility, hyperactivity, loss of coordination

        3.   Patient, family knowledge deficit related to: medication effects or side effects, safety needs

    E.   Planning and Intervention

        1.   For phenothiazine toxicity:

            a)   Stop phenothiazine

            b)   Benztropine mesylate (Cogentin®), trihexyphenidyl (Artane®, Tremin®), diphenhydramine (Benadryl®)

        2.   For akathisia (inability to sit still, pacing, agitation, restless movements):

            a)   Benzodiazepines (lorazepam (Ativan®), diazepam (Valium®))

            b)   OR beta-blockers (propranolol (Inderal®))

3. For dystonia, slow, retarded movements: physical or occupational therapy may be an adjunct if appropriate according to patient's place in the disease process, trajectory

4. In elderly, or others who may have sensitivity to anticholinergics: amantadine (Symmetrel®)

5. Review of symptoms being treated with medication that may cause EPS; if symptoms remain present, discussion with medical team regarding alternative medications to control

F. Patient/family education

1. Stopping medication that may be contributing to EPS

2. Expected medication effects and potential side effects

3. Monitoring patient activity; safety in ambulation

G. Evaluate for effectiveness of interventions, specifically

1. Effect of medication change on EPS symptoms

2. Patient/family compliance, comfort with new medications

3. Control of symptoms

H. Revise plan according to findings from ongoing evaluations, changes in patient status or family needs

XVI. Hematologic Symptoms

A. Definitions

1. **Hemorrhage:** excessive bleeding

2. **Clotting:** systemic response to disease or medication that initiates coagulation cascade causing clotting

3. **Cytopenia:** reduction in bone marrow blood cell components, which can precipitate a systemic response

    a) Neutropenia: reduction in white blood cells; decreases patient's ability to respond to infection

    b) Thrombocytopenia: reduction in platelets; increases potential for frank, uncontrolled bleeding

    c) Anemias: reduction in production or maturation of red blood cells; low hemoglobin; decreased oxygen carrying cells; increased dyspnea, fatigue

    d) Pancytopenia: reduction in all blood cells

B. Possible etiologies

1. Initiating coagulation cascade: deep vein thrombosis (DVT)

2. Immunologic processes (AIDS), drug-induced processes, prosthetic cardiac valves, veno-occlusive liver disease initiating coagulation cascade: hemorrhage, disseminated intravascular coagulopathy (DIC)

3. Chemotherapy, radiotherapy or disorders of spleen: thrombocytopenia, pancytopenia

4. Tumor erosion of blood vessels: hemorrhage

5. Pulmonary embolism (PE)

C. Assess for:

1. Review medical history and current medications for potential hematology problems

2. Review current medications, foods, herbals for interactions with anticoagulant therapy

3. For DIC: petechiae, ecchymosis, oozing blood from mucous membranes, body orifices, puncture sites, signs of decreased perfusion to brain, kidneys, gastrointestinal, cardiovascular and peripheral vascular systems, lungs

4. For DVT: possible peripheral phlebitis, noting vascular access devices, streaking, erythema, heat over vein

5. For pulmonary embolism: sudden onset dyspnea

6. For thrombocytopenia: periorbital petechiae, epistaxis, gingival bleeding, blood-streaked sputum, emesis, urine or stool; acute shortness of breath, inspiratory pain, vaginal bleeding, petechiae, ecchymosis, joint pain, change in mental status, paresthesias

7. Patient/family understanding of and coping with changes in blood clotting response or pancytopenia; non-pharmacologic therapies, safety

D. Potential Diagnoses

1. Injury risk due to altered clotting patterns related to etiology

2. Infection risk due to neutropenia and body's reduced ability to control or fight infection

3. Patient/family knowledge deficit related to expected medication effects or side effects, safety needs, e.g. injury or infection

4. Medication risk related to anticoagulant therapy and other medications, herbals, foods

E. Plan and Intervention: treat underlying problem if appropriate

1. For DVT: anticoagulant therapy; monitor for other medications, foods and herbals that may interfere with anticoagulant therapy; antiembolic stockings

2. For PE: anticoagulant therapy; monitor other medications, food and herbals that may interfere with anticoagulant therapy; antiembolic stockings, treatment of dyspnea, pain

3. For Thrombocytopenia:

    a) If palliative care: bleeding precautions, platelet transfusion for platelets <10,000, if appropriate

    b) If hospice: bleeding precautions, treat bleeding with compression, other non-pharmacologic interventions

4. For DIC: replenish clotting factors, e.g. platelets, fresh frozen plasma, antithrombin factor in palliative care; patient should be in an acute care facility for ongoing monitoring during therapy

5. For neutropenia: institute precautions against introduction of bacteria, infections to patient

6. Patient, family support, instruction, reassurance during bleeding and in anticipation of bleed

F.   Patient/family education

1. Bleeding precautions:

   a)   Soft toothbrush and gentle motions for tooth brushing

   b)   Care when using eating utensils

   c)   Rinses for mouth

   d)   No suppositories

   e)   Safety in ambulation; prevent falls, injury

   f)   Use electric razor rather than straight razor

2. For active bleed: long pressure for active bleed; use of dark towels; whom to call

3. For PE: elevate head of bed for dyspnea; palliative oxygen if needed

4. For DVT: use of antiembolic stockings applied before ambulation; expected anticoagulation medicine effects and side effects

5. Medicines, food and herbals that can affect anticoagulation including Vitamin E, theophylline, tegretol, dilantin, Vitamin K (especially high in dark green vegetables)

6. For neutropenia: regular and frequent hand washing; plants, flowers not in direct proximity; support of family in encouraging visitors with colds, illness to visit when they are well

7. Review, rehearse with patient and family the steps to take if bleeding begins

G.   Evaluate

1. Effectiveness of medical therapies

2. Patient compliance with anticoagulant therapy; for therapeutic PTT/PT (partial thromboplastin time/prothrombin time)

3. Safety in ambulation

4. Patient/family understanding regarding disease process, safety, expected medicine effects and potential side effects

H.   Revise plan according to findings from ongoing evaluations, changes in patient status or family needs

XVII. Hiccoughs

A. Definition: an involuntary contraction of the diaphragm, followed by rapid closure of the glottis

B. Possible etiologies

1. Gastric distention: impaired gastric motility, excessive gas

2. Central nervous system: neoplasm, stroke, multiple sclerosis, ventriculoperitoneal shunts, atriovenous malformations, hydrocephalus, lesions from head trauma

3. Peripheral nervous system: irritation of phrenic or vagus nerve

4. Tumors of the neck, lung, mediastinum

5. Chest surgery or trauma

6. Respiratory disorders: pulmonary edema, pneumonia, bronchitis, asthma, COPD

7. Gastrointestinal disorders: esophagitis or esophageal obstruction, gastritis, peptic ulcer disease, gastric cancer, pancreatitis, pancreatic cancer, bowel obstruction, cholelithiasis/cholecystitis

8. Renal/hepatic disorders

9. Metabolic Disorders: Uremia, hypocalcemia, hyponatremia

10. Infectious Disease: Sepsis, influenza, herpes zoster, malaria, tuberculosis

11. Pharmacologic Agents: General anesthesia, IV corticosteroids, barbiturates, benzodiazepines, diazepam, chlordiazepoxide

12. Psychogenic: Stress, excitement, grief reactions, anorexia, personality disorders

C. Assess for:

1. Etiology of hiccoughs related to medical/psychological history and/or medication usage

2. Associated signs and symptoms (underlying disease process, etc.)

3. Severity and duration of current episode and previous episodes

4. Relationship of hiccoughs to sleep: hiccoughs that stop during sleep suggest a psychogenic cause

5. Patient/family concerns and knowledge: Are the hiccoughs troublesome? Does anything help to alleviate hiccoughs?

D. Diagnoses

1. Alteration in comfort related to hiccoughs

2. Risk for fluid/nutritional deficit related to dysphagia secondary to hiccoughs

3. Risk for sleep pattern disturbance related to hiccoughs

4. Patient/family knowledge deficit related to etiology and treatment of hiccoughs

E.   Planning and Intervention: Etiology of hiccoughs can guide intervention plan (i.e., possible reversal of metabolic disorders)

1.   Non-pharmacologic Interventions: Before suggesting non-pharmacologic techniques, assure patient safety and do not suggest techniques that may be harmful, depending upon diagnosis

   a)   Nasopharyngeal stimulation

   (1)   Swallowing one teaspoon of granulated sugar

   (2)   Lifting uvula with a spoon or cotton-tip applicator

   (3)   Gargling with water

   (4)   Biting on a lemon

   (5)   Swallowing crushed ice

   b)   Interference with normal respiratory function

   (1)   Induction of sneezing or coughing

   (2)   Re-breathing into paper bag

   (3)   Breath holding or hyperventilation

   c)   Etiology related to gastric distention

   (1)   Nasogastric suction

   (2)   Gastric lavage

   d)   Complementary therapies:

   (1)   Hypnosis and/or behavior modification

   (2)   Acupuncture

   e)   Distraction

2.   Pharmacologic Techniques

   a)   If etiology is related to gastric distention:

   (1)   Simethicone before or after meals

   (2)   Metoclopramide alone or with simethicone before meals

   b)   Peppermint oil relaxes lower esophageal sphincter and is useful for hiccoughs related to esophageal disorders; has opposing action with metoclopramide

   c)   Baclofen if simethicone and metoclopramide fail

   d)   Calcium channel blockers, e.g., nifedipine

   e)   Chlorpromazine 25–50 mg tid effective for uremic etiology, but useful in other etiologies as well; postural hypotension a significant side effect, especially when used IV

f)   Anticonvulsants: carbamazepine, phenytoin, and valproic acid

g)   Nebulized lidocaine (3 cm^3 of 4% topical lidocaine nebulized in a standard small-particle nebulizer)

3.   Invasive Techniques

a)   Phrenic nerve interruption with bupivicaine or surgery

b)   Pacing electrodes for direct phrenic nerve or diaphragmatic stimulation

F.   Patient/Family Education

1.   Explain etiology and instruct in ways to treat

2.   Explain appropriate, safe non-pharmacological techniques that are realistic for individual patient

3.   Expected medication effects and side effects

4.   Post-surgical care, if indicated

G.   Evaluate

1.   Effectiveness of non-pharmacological techniques and/or medication

2.   Control of hiccoughs

3.   Patient/family understanding of regimen

H.   Revise plan according to findings from ongoing evaluations, changes in patient status or family needs

XVIII.   Impaired Mobility, Fatigue, Lethargy, Weakness

A.   Definitions

1.   Impaired Mobility: a loss or abnormality of function due to physiological, anatomical, psychological or fatigue factors

2.   Fatigue: an overwhelming sustained sense of exhaustion with decreased capacity for physical or mental activity[8]

3.   Lethargy: a condition of functional torpor or sluggishness; stupor[8]

4.   Weakness: a subjective term to indicate a lack of strength as compared to what patient feels is normal

B.   Potential etiologies

1.   Disease process:

a)   Sudden onset of weakness or impaired mobility: consider neurologic deficit, e.g., spinal cord compression or other CNS tumor effects; sudden generalized weakness may be adrenal failure or septicemia

b)   Chronic disease: chronic obstructive pulmonary disease (COPD), congestive heart failure (CHF)

    c)   Tumor infiltration of bone marrow

    d)   Liver disease with coagulopathy

    e)   Hypothyroidism; adrenal or hormonal insufficiencies (including chemical and hormonal response to tumor)

    f)   Uremia: related to kidney failure, tumor, or use of nephrotoxic drugs

    g)   Metabolic: hypercalcemia from metastatic disease, parathyroid disease

2. Uncontrolled pain or other symptoms, anemia, blood loss

3. Some medications or therapies may contribute to lethargy, weakness: beta blockers, antihistamines, benzodiazepines, phenothiazines, zidovudine, myelosuppressive chemotherapy, radiation therapy

4. Nutritional deficiencies:

    a)   Decreased iron, B-12, folate

    b)   Anorexia, nausea, vomiting, weight loss

    c)   GI malabsorption

5. Infectious processes:

    a)   AIDS-related infections

    b)   Pneumonia

    c)   Urinary tract infections

6. Emotional factors: depression, anxiety, sleep disturbance, psychological or spiritual distress, family distress

7. Environmental factors: multiple sensory stimuli (noise, lights, odors)

C.   Assess for etiology, which will determine intervention plan

1. Thorough history

    a)   Onset, history of or change in functional status

    b)   Patient's own description of fatigue, weakness: does it relate to activity? Is it constant? Intermittent?

    c)   Effect of lethargy, fatigue, weakness on quality of life scores[15]

    d)   Patient's place on disease trajectory of end-stage or terminal illness

2. Symptom management: review adequacy of pain control and management of other debilitating symptoms (including nausea, vomiting, dyspnea, anxiety, depression)

3. Current medications for appropriate use and dose for patient's current weight

4. Psychosocial factors:

    a)   Sleep, rest disturbance

    b)   Depression, anxiety component

    c)   Unresolved psychological or spiritual issues or distress

5. Family, caregiver perceptions and impact of patient's fatigue; understanding of disease process

6. Infectious or disease process

7. Dyspnea if anemic

D. Potential diagnoses

1. Activity alteration from fatigue due to: (etiology)

2. Self-care deficit related to activity intolerance

3. Risk for altered nutritional, functional status due to activity disturbance

4. Patient, family knowledge deficit of non-pharmacologic interventions, expected medication effects, side effects

5. Impaired physical mobility related to: [injury, potential for injury, pain]

6. Alteration in perceived quality of life from fatigue

7. Altered self-image and role disturbance related to change in functional abilities and endurance

E. Planning and Interventions: etiology of fatigue, impaired mobility, lethargy and weakness will determine intervention plan

1. Patient's place on disease trajectory for end-stage or terminal illness, wishes and advance directives will influence treatment decisions

2. Treat specific underlying causes as appropriate

   a) If anemia: based on classification of anemia, consider treatment of cause

   b) If endocrine disorder: determine appropriate therapy

   c) If medication-induced (iatrogenic):

      (1) Consider tapering or discontinuing medicine

      (2) If opioid induced, fatigue may resolve when patient develops tolerance (usually 48–72 hours after dose increase)

      (3) If opioid induced lethargy continues and other etiologies have been ruled out and is unacceptable to the patient/family, consider adding methylphenidate 5 mg po in the A.M. and at noon to combat sedation and to improve appetite and mood[16.] Titrate if not effective.

3. For depression, anxiety: see Chapter VI, Section VI, C.3

4. Non-pharmacologic interventions:

   a) Balance activities with rest

   b) Hospital bed and other equipment as needed to decrease exertional fatigue

   c) Set realistic goals for ADL's and other activities

   d) Exercise, physical and occupational therapy as indicated, if tolerated

   e) Increase team services for personal care as needed

F.   Patient and Family Education

1.   Instruct regarding balancing activities and rest

2.   Set activity priorities: e.g. a bedside commode may help patient to conserve the energy used walking to the bathroom for other activities

3.   Expected medication effects and potential side effects especially as they may contribute to fatigue or sedation

4.   Educate family of hospice patient in terminal phase regarding end-stage disease process and encourage setting of realistic expectations

5.   For the palliative care patient who is not in terminal phase of disease process, discourage prolonged bedrest or excessive inactivity explaining possible adverse physical (deep vein thrombosis [DVT], pulmonary embolism [PE], pneumonia, increased weakness) and emotional (depression, decreased motivation, social isolation) effects

G.   Evaluate

1.   Effectiveness of interventions and ability of the caregivers to provide care

2.   Improvement in activity tolerance

3.   Patient for signs of disease progression

4.   Patient, family understanding, coping with ongoing fatigue, balancing activities, prioritizing to accomplish essential or preferred activities

5.   Further adjustments in team visit frequency to assist in personal care as needed

H.   Revise plan according to findings from ongoing evaluations, changes in patient status or family needs

XIX. Increased Intracranial Pressure (ICP)

A.   Definition: increase in the pressure within the cranial cavity due to increased volume of fluid or mass

B.   Possible etiologies

1.   Space occupying tumors, metastatic lesions with surrounding edema

2.   Intracranial hemorrhage

3.   Inflammatory process: abscess, encephalitis, meningitis

4.   Obstruction of CSF flow

C.   Assess for:

1.   Sudden unanticipated changes in patient condition with signs of increased ICP: new headache, vomiting, changed respiratory pattern, decreased motor function, lethargy to altered mental status, increased restlessness, agitation, blurred vision

2.   Documentation of possible etiologies of increased ICP in past medical history

3.   Patient and family anxiety, ability to cope with changes in condition; knowledge and/or understanding of presenting changes, disease process, treatment options

D. Potential Diagnoses

1. Altered mental status due to increased ICP

2. Cerebral alteration related to increased ICP

3. Patient and family knowledge deficit related to: disease process, current symptom changes, coping strategies

E. Planning and Interventions

1. Treat underlying etiology if appropriate

2. Steroids to reduce edema/inflammation

3. Anticonvulsant if seizure activity

4. Palliative radiotherapy when appropriate

5. Analgesia for headache

    a) Keep in mind that opioids can mildly increase ICP due to vasodilatation effects and mild respiratory depression

    b) Tramadol (Ultram®) should not be used in increased ICP as it may lower seizure threshold[17]

6. Non-pharmacologic measures: head of bed 45–60 degrees, darkened room, reduce external stimuli in environment, calm presence

F. Patient/family education

1. Reassurance and instruction regarding possible cause for changes in patient condition

2. Review goals of therapy to reduce intracranial pressure symptoms and increase patient comfort and safety

3. Preparation for changes that may indicate advancement of disease and decline of patient condition; support of family/caregiver goals, needs

4. Consider transfer of home hospice patient to inpatient hospice facility or palliative care facility bed if management is beyond physical, emotional capacity of family or caregiver

G. Evaluate

1. Effectiveness of medications, patient comfort and relief, reduction of increased ICP symptoms

2. Patient/family understanding, coping, anxiety related to current symptoms, plan

H. Revise plan according to findings from ongoing evaluations, changes in patient status or family needs

XX. Myoclonus

A. Definition: twitching or brief spasm of a muscle or muscle group

B. Possible etiologies

1. High dose opioid therapy

2. Metabolic derangement, e.g. uremia

3. Inflammatory or degenerative CNS diseases, e.g. Jakob-Creutzfeld, subacute sclerosing panencephalitis, end-stage Alzheimer's

4. Hypercalcemia from osteoblastic activity of bone metastases

C. Assess for:

1. Onset, duration of myoclonus and its impact on patient and patient functional status

2. Interruption of sleep, rest

3. Patient, family anxiety related to myocolonic jerking

4. Patient/family understanding of disease process, medication effects and side effects

5. Potential etiology which will direct intervention plan:

   a) If opioid-induced, evaluate adjuvant use that would allow for pain to be managed using a reduced opioid dose or rotate opioids. Dose can often be decreased because of incomplete cross tolerance.

   b) If hypercalcemia, evaluate patient's place on the disease trajectory

6. Patient safety if ambulatory or if bed bound due to uncontrolled muscular jerking movements

D. Potential Diagnoses

1. Alteration in metabolic status related to: uremia, hypercalcemia, etc.

2. Alteration in functional status due to impairment of neuro-musculoskeletal system

3. Disturbance of sleep and rest pattern due to myoclonus

4. Patient, family knowledge deficit regarding: medication effects, disease process, safety precautions

E. Planning and intervention: Etiology of myoclonus will direct intervention plan

1. Non-pharmacologic adjunct therapies including local heat, gentle massage, relaxation

2. If hypercalcemia etiology:

   a) In palliative care, may consider pamidronate (Aredia®) q 3–4 weeks to decrease serum calcium

   b) In hospice, supplementary hydration (IV or PO) may decrease serum calcium and relieve symptoms

3. If opioid-induced, consider adjuvant medicines for the specific type of pain (neuropathic or bone) at the most appropriate dose that may allow reduction in opioid dose or rotate opioids

4. If unable to treat underlying metabolic or degenerative disorder because of advanced stage of disease, patient/family wishes, treat symptoms with clonazepam, valproic acid

5. Occasionally muscle relaxants provide benefit:

    a) Diazepam (Valium®)

    b) Baclofen (Lioresal®)

    c) Cyclobenzaprine (Flexeril®)

        (1) Cyclobenzaprine should be used cautiously in elderly or debilitated patients

        (2) Increases side effects of other medications often taken by the elderly and has side effects that can contribute to conditions often already present such as CHF, glaucoma, etc.

6. If night cramps only, quinine sulfate at bedtime

F. Patient and family education

1. Discuss possible etiologies and recommended interventions

2. Expected medication effects and potential side effects

3. Non-pharmacologic methods of intervention: heat, gentle massage, relaxation to decrease anxiety

G. Evaluate for effectiveness of interventions, specifically

1. Decrease in or resolution of myoclonus

2. Maintenance of effective pain control

3. Patient/family understanding of instructions, recommendations

4. Patient safety

H. Revise plan according to findings from ongoing evaluations, changes in patient status or family needs

XXI. Nausea and Vomiting

    A. Definitions

        1. Nausea is a subjectively perceived, stomach discomfort ranging from stomach awareness to the conscious recognition of the need to vomit

        2. Vomiting is the expelling of stomach contents through the mouth

    B. Possible etiologies[18, 11, 4]

        1. Fluid and electrolyte imbalances (hypercalcemia, hyponatremia, uremia, dehydration)

        2. Gastrointestinal disorders (pressure due to tumor, organomegaly; distention; ascites; esophageal, gastrointestinal, and hepatic malignancies; constipation; bowel obstruction; GI stasis)

        3. Other physiologic disorders (oral thrush; cough; pain; high fever)

        4. Neurologic disorders (primary and metastatic CNS tumors, increased intracranial pressure)

        5. Renal failure

        6. Vestibular (tumors and bone metastases at skull base; motion sickness)

        7. Chemical (radiation, medications such as chemotherapy, antibiotics, aspirin, iron, steroids, digoxin, expectorants, NSAIDs, opioids, theophylline)

        8. Psychogenic (anxiety; anticipatory nausea and vomiting; fear)

        9. Adverse response to certain foods especially high fat content

      10. Adverse response to certain drugs e.g. increase in opioids

    C. Assess for:

        1. History of the onset of nausea and vomiting and concomitant symptoms i.e., heartburn, constipation, excessive thirst and other symptoms that can indicate etiology

        2. Pattern of nausea: When does nausea occur? Are there contributing factors?

        3. If possible, assess vomitus for volume, color, odor, presence of blood (vomitus with fecal odor or fecal material indicates possible bowel obstruction; coffee ground emesis indicates old blood, whereas fresh blood indicates current hemorrhage)

        4. Abdominal assessment: pain or cramps, bowel sounds, distention

        5. Oropharynx for infection (thrush) or presence of tenacious sputum

        6. Neurologic signs of increased intracranial pressure

        7. Other factors that could trigger nausea response: malodorous wounds, pain, fear, anxiety

    D. Potential diagnoses

        1. Nausea related to metabolic disorders, tumor pressure, therapies, neurosensory disorders, or anxiety

        2. Risk for fluid volume deficit related to nausea and vomiting

3. Risk for altered nutrition due to intake less than body requirements related to inability to eat or keep food down secondary to nausea and vomiting

4. Patient/family knowledge deficit related to etiology and treatment of nausea and vomiting

E. Planning and Intervention: Etiology of nausea and vomiting may guide interventions

1. Modify diet to decrease nausea

    a) Bland foods that patient enjoys, e.g., baked potatoes, soft fruits, yogurt, soft drinks, crackers or dry toast, clear liquids such as Popsicles, Jell-O, sports drinks, foods without aggressive odors, non-gassy foods

    b) Cold or room temperature foods are often better tolerated than warm foods due to less odor

    c) Serve small, frequent meals

    d) Avoid fatty, greasy, spicy or very sweet foods

2. Correct reversible causes of nausea, including cough, hypercalcemia, increased intracranial pressure

3. Keep the patient cool; place a fan in the room or open a window to circulate air

4. Keep patient's head elevated

5. Medication regimen (See Table 3) should be prescribed according to etiology of nausea[4, 19]

    a) A prokinetic agent (metoclopramide (Reglan®)) can be used for delayed gastric emptying (do not use in bowel obstruction)

    b) Butyrophenones, i.e. haloperidol (Haldol®) or droperidol for opioid-induced nausea (nausea related to opioid initiation generally resolves within one week)

    c) An antihistamine (meclizine (Antivert®), dimenhydramine) can be used for bowel obstruction or other visceral irritation (liver metastases, constipation, etc.), disturbances in the vestibular system (vertigo, motion sickness), pharyngeal stimulation (tenacious sputum, oral thrush), or increased intracranial pressure (which can also be treated with a glucocorticoid such as dexamethasone)

    d) Anticholinergics (scopolamine patches, hydroxyzine (Atarax®)) are used primarily for increased intracranial pressure and vestibular disturbances

    e) Nausea related to disturbances in the chemoreceptor trigger zone (CTZ) (usually due to metabolic disorders, medications, and toxins produced from GI tumors, infection, poisoning, etc.), can be treated by discontinuing offending medication if possible, and utilizing drugs which act on the CTZ (haloperidol, metoclopramide, phenothiazines)

    f) Nausea related to emetogenic chemotherapy can be treated with 5-HT$_3$ serotonin receptor antagonists (ondansetron (Zofran®), granisetron (Kytril®))

    g) Nausea related to anxiety and fear can be treated with antihistamines or anticholinergics

6. Oral hygiene before and after meals

F.   Patient/Family Education

1.   Explain etiology and treatment course of nausea and vomiting

2.   Explain effects of medication and possible side effects

3.   Explain non-pharmacologic measures to treat nausea and vomiting, including diet, oral hygiene, etc.

G.   Evaluate

1.   Effectiveness of interventions and patient/family teaching (are patient/family satisfied with outcome?)

2.   Medication effectiveness and presence of side effects

3.   Patient/family understanding of treatment measures

H.   Revise plan according to findings from ongoing evaluations, changes in patient status, or family needs

Table 3: Management of Nausea/Vomiting*

Syndrome Pathway(s)**	Causes	Clinical Features	Antiemetic Management	Adjuvant
S Gastric stasis and gastric outflow obstruction **P** Vomiting center, GI tract	Anticholinergic drugs, autonomic failure, ascites, hepatomegaly, tumor infiltration, peptic ulcer, gastritis	Epigastric fullness and discomfort. Early satiety. Flatulence, hiccup, acid reflux and gastric regurgitation. Large volume emesis which may contain undigested food. Nausea often relieved by vomiting	Prokinetic Metoclopramide 10–20 mg tid po 40–80 mg sq infusion/ 24 hours	Dietary advice. Paracentesis for ascites. Simethicone for flatulence. Steroid therapy may be used to improve the dysfunction induced by tumor infiltration of nerve plexuses. For total obstruction a venting gastrostomy or surgical bypass may be considered. H_2 blocker or proton pump inhibitor. Review drug regimen.
S Stretch/ irritation of visceral and GI serosa **P** Vomiting center, GI tract	Liver metastases, ureteric obstruction, tumor, constipation, bowel obstruction, lymph nodes	Pain is often a feature. Colic. Altered bowel habits. Nausea. Vomiting of fecal fluid in obstruction.	Antihistamine *Diphenhydramine* 25–50 mg tid or qid po/IM/IV *Promethazine* 12.5–25 mg tid or qid po/IM/IV/PR *Hydroxyzine* 25–100 mg tid or qid po/IM	Relieve the cause, e.g., constipation with stimulant laxatives and enemas as required. Steroid therapy for the reduction of peri-tumor edema

* Adapted with permission from: Campbell, T. & Hately, J. (2000). The management of nausea and vomiting in advanced cancer. *International Journal of Palliative Nursing, 6*(1): pp. 18–20, 22–25.

** Editor's Note: **S** = Syndrome, **P** = Pathway(s).

Table 3: Management of Nausea/Vomiting (cont)

Syndrome Pathway(s)	Causes	Clinical Features	Antiemetic Management	Adjuvant
S Raised intracranial pressure/ meningism **P** Vomiting center	Cerebral tumor, intracranial tumor, intracranial bleeding, infiltration of meninges by tumor, skull metastases, cerebral infection	Neurological signs, e.g. cyclovir, drowsiness, dizziness, headache, nausea and/or vomiting, vomiting may be projectile in nature	Antihistamine *Diphenhydramine* 25–50 mg tid or qid po/IM/IV *Promethazine* 12.5–25 mg tid or qid po/IM/IV/PR *Hydroxyzine* 25–100 mg tid or qid po/IM Anticholinergic *Scopolamine Transdermal patch* q 3 days	High dose steroids may reduce cerebral edema and/or tumor mass
S Pharyngeal stimulation **P** Vomiting center	Tenacious sputum not easily expectorated, infection *(candida)*	Retching	Antihistamine *Diphenhydramine* 25–50 mg tid or qid po/IM/IV *Promethazine* 12.5–25 mg tid or qid po/IM/IV/PR *Hydroxyzine* 25–100 mg tid or qid po/IM	Treat the cause. Saline nebulizers. Antibiotics. Antifungal therapy.
S Esophageal obstruction **P** Vomiting center	Tumor, odynophagia (painful swallowing), functional dysphagia, *candida*	Regurgitation, dysphagia	Anticholinergic Will help to reduce saliva and secretions *Scopolamine Transdermal patch* q 3 days	Radiotherapy, brachiotherapy, laser therapy, high dose steroids, self-expanding stent, Celestin or Atkinson tube, Surgery (not for patients with metastatic spread)
S Anxiety **P** Vomiting center	Psychological and emotional distress, anticipatory emesis associated with chemotherapy	Nausea, waves of nausea and vomiting, distraction may relieve symptoms	Antihistamine or Anticholinergics if required	Address the anxiety with psychological techniques. Relaxation. Benzodiazepines. Ensure adequate pain control.

XXII. Paresthesia and Neuropathy

A. Definitions

1. **Paresthesia:** a sensation of numbness, prickling or tingling; heightened sensitivity

2. **Neuropathy:** any disease of the nerves; may include sensory loss, muscle weakness and atrophy and decreased deep tendon reflexes

B. Possible etiologies

1. Central and peripheral nerve lesions

2. Direct damage to peripheral and autonomic nerves

3. Metabolic and vascular changes of diabetes mellitus

4. Chemical or drug-induced: e.g. chemotherapy, isoniazid, alcohol

5. Amputation, AIDS, Vitamin B-12 deficiency

6. Tumor invasion with pressure on nerves or plexuses

7. Spinal cord compression (considered an oncologic emergency)

C. Assess for:

1. Sudden loss of sensation, motor function of lower extremities with or without loss of bladder or bowel control; **MAY INDICATE SPINAL CORD COMPRESSION WHICH IS A MEDICAL EMERGENCY.** Most common signs of pending cord compression is escalating back pain with or without bladder changes and before lower extremity weakness, worse when lying down, improved when standing. Amount of neurological deficit patient presents with is usually amount left with following treatment, therefore early recognition is imperative.

2. Location and degree of numbness: patient's subjective descriptions of pain or sensation assist in determining etiology

3. Patient's course in the diseases process/trajectory for assistance in intervention planning

4. Patient safety in ambulation, ADLs

5. Patient/family understanding of cause of sudden change in sensation or motor function, need for safety in ambulation/ADLs, understanding of treatment options

D. Potential Diagnoses

1. Alteration in comfort related to peripheral sensory and neuropathic changes

2. Safety risk related to alteration in sensation

3. Patient/family knowledge deficit related to safety needs, medication effects, treatment options

4. Compromised patient, family coping related to uncontrolled pain

E. Planning and Intervention: Determining patient's course in disease process, trajectory will facilitate planning in the event of spinal cord compression

1. If patient is in advanced stage of disease (weak, bed bound, poor nutritional status), symptom management may be appropriate option, i.e., steroids to decrease edema around cord; neuroleptic analgesia, opioids

2. If patient is ambulatory, active and able to participate in self-care, palliative radiotherapy and steroids may provide significant benefit for quality of life

3. Tricyclic antidepressants (TCA's) are appropriate adjuvant analgesics to opioids for neuropathic pain (see Chapter IV, Section III. A. 2. d.)

   a) Titrate dose every few days based upon the patient's response

   b) Therapeutic levels achieved in 3–7 days

4. Anticonvulsants can be considered for neuropathic pain:

   a) If gabapentin: start low. Dose can be titrated to 3600 mg daily maximum (in divided doses) for therapeutic effect

   b) If carbamazepine or phenytoin: monitor for effect and for drug interaction (Monitor CBC–ADE is pancytopenic)

5. Appropriate bowel regimen if patient has decreased activity, is bed bound or has lost sensation in rectum

6. Foley catheter for urinary retention

7. Condom or Foley catheter for urinary incontinence if this causes skin irritation, patient anxiety and if patient/caregiver agree

8. Increase assistance with ADLs in home as indicated for patient personal needs and safety

F. Patient/family education

1. Expected medication effects and possible side effects

   a) Continue TCA's regularly

      (1) It takes 3–7 days to become therapeutic for neuropathic pain

      (2) Give at night, which might aid in sleeping and reduce daytime sedation

   b) Prepare patient/family to expect that gabapentin may cause sedation when initiated or dose increased

   c) Carbamazepine may cause dizziness, drowsiness, anorexia and nausea

   d) Phenytoin may cause ataxia, diplopia. dizziness, drowsiness

2. Safety needs when ambulating related to decreased sensation, motor ability and medication effects

G. Evaluate for effectiveness of interventions, specifically

    1.   Compliance with medication regimen

    2.   Effectiveness of medication and any side effects

    3.   Return of sensation, function

    4.   Safety needs/issues

H. Revise plan according to findings from ongoing evaluations, changes in patient status or family needs

XXIII. Seizures

A. Definitions: usually intermittent tonic, clonic movements; convulsions caused by a large number of neurons discharging abnormally[20]

    1.   Primary (generalized) involving large parts of the brain and including grand mal and petit mal types

    2.   Focal (partial) involving specific regions of the brain with symptoms reflecting the location of the disturbance

B. Possible etiologies[20]

    1.   Brain infarct, primary brain tumor or brain metastases, cerebral abscess, brain infection in HIV and AIDS

    2.   Increased intracranial pressure (may be associated with SIADH in some cancer patients)

    3.   Pre-existing seizure disorder

    4.   Medications (metabolites from normeperidine and propoxyphene) and their preservatives (sodium bisulfite); medications that lower seizure threshold include phenothiazines, butyrophenones, tricyclic antidepressants

    5.   Infection, stroke, hemorrhage, oxygen deprivation, paraneoplastic syndromes

    6.   Metabolic instability (hyponatremia, hypercalcemia, hypomagnesemia, hypoxemia, hypoglycemia)

    7.   Drug toxicity, drug withdrawal

C. Assess for:

    1.   Acutely seizing patient: intervene with first intervention below

    2.   Underlying etiology reviewing medical history, disease process, current medications, history of trauma or recent fall, differentiate from myoclonus

    3.   Question patient and/or family to determine onset and type of seizure, presence of aura, headache, nausea and projectile vomiting

    4.   Drug levels if previously taking anticonvulsants; EEG may be warranted

    5.   Patient/family coping with seizure activity, their understanding of patient protection/safety during seizure, medication effects and side effects

D. **Potential Diagnoses**

1. Safety precautions (e.g. risk for falls) for seizures from: etiology

2. Potential risk for medication toxicity or withdrawal side effects

    a) Dexamethasone is commonly given to those with seizure disorder; interaction between this drug and phenytoin is problematic

    b) Phenytoin increases bioavailability of dexamethasone and dexamethasone inhibits metabolism of phenytoin

    c) Steroids must not be suddenly stopped—seizures may occur

3. Metabolic impairment related to: hyponatremia, hypercalcemia, hypomagnesemia, hypoxia, hypoglycemia

4. Patient, family knowledge deficit related to: etiology, disease process, medication effects/side effects, safety

E. **Planning and Intervention**

1. For actively seizing patient:

    a) Assess airway, breathing, circulation and ensure adequate airway

    b) Protect patient from harm and ensure safety

    c) Model calm demeanor

    d) Medical therapy may include:

        (1) IV lorazepam (Ativan®)

        (2) Diazepam enema, IV diazepam (Valium®)

        (3) Fosphenytoin IV (Cerebyx®)

        (4) Initiation of phenytoin (Dilantin®), carbamazepine (Tegretol®), valproic acid (Depakene®) or phenobarbital[20]

2. Determine potentially treatable etiologies:

    a) Hypoglycemia: glucose PO/IV or glucagon SQ as indicated

    b) Hyponatremia: fluid restriction, IV NaCl, adjustment of diuretics

    c) Hypercalcemia: increase fluids PO/IV, pamidronate may be appropriate depending on disease trajectory

    d) Hypoxemia: supplemental O_2; further evaluation of this etiology

    e) Hypomagnesemia: supplemental magnesium

    f) Infectious process (cerebral abscess, encephalitis, meningitis): antibiotics as indicated and according to patient's place on disease trajectory and advance directives

    g) Substance abuse: support withdrawal, consult substance withdrawal specialist

F.   Patient/family education

1.   Anticipate potential for seizure activity and prepare family for patient safety, preemptive interventions, whom to call

2.   Calmly rehearse, review caregiver interventions

3.   Expected medication effects and potential side effects

G.   Evaluate

1.   Effectiveness of seizure management interventions

2.   Family preparedness and coping

3.   Patient safety

4.   Medication effects and side effects

5.   Blood draws to monitor levels of medications such as phenytoin

    a)   Phenytoin has a narrow therapeutic range, and drug interactions may lead to alterations in its plasma concentration

    b)   This may result in either phenytoin intoxication or in decreased effectiveness of the drug[21]

H.   Revise plan according to findings from ongoing evaluations, changes in patient status or family needs

XXIV. Urinary Incontinence/Retention

A.   Definition: the inability to control urination

B.   Possible etiologies

1.   Urge incontinence: urge to void sensed, but cannot control urine flow long enough to reach toilet

    a)   Due to bladder irritation such as infection, tumor, radiation, or chemotherapy

    b)   Nervous system damage: Spinal cord lesions (neurogenic bladder), stroke, multiple sclerosis, Parkinson's, Alzheimer's

    c)   Decreased mobility or difficulty reaching the toilet in time

2.   Stress incontinence: leakage of urine when intra-abdominal pressure is raised.

    a)   Damage or dysfunction of bladder sphincter due to:

        (1)   Tumor infiltration in GU system or CNS or spinal cord lesions

        (2)   Multiparity or post-menopausal changes in women

3.   Overflow incontinence: bladder unable to empty normally

    a)   Bladder outlet obstruction due to fecal mass, tumor, calculi, prostatic hypertrophy

    b)   Detrusor muscle failure due to anticholinergic drugs, CNS lesions, or debility and confusion

4. Functional incontinence: an involuntary or unpredictable passage of urine with no impairment of the GU tract

    a) Cognitive dysfunction: Depression leading to self-neglect, confusion, excessive sedation

    b) Mobility or functional problems: Immobility, unable to undress, inaccessible toilet facilities, final stage of illness

5. Many drugs can lead to any of the aforementioned urinary incontinence problems:

    a) Diuretics increase volume and frequency

    b) Sedatives decrease awareness of need to void, as well as decrease bladder contraction and outlet resistance

    c) Anticholinergics decrease bladder contraction

    d) Antiparkinson drugs increase outlet resistance

6. Metabolic disorders: hypercalcemia

7. Atonic bladder: No awareness of bladder fullness or urgency

    a) Diabetic neuropathy

    b) Spinal cord lesions or cord compression

    c) Neurologic dysfunction

8. Fistula

C. **Assess for:**

1. History, including nature and duration of symptoms, medications, recent treatments for cancer

2. Physical exam: bladder distention, perineal swelling, fecal impaction, simple neurologic exam (including sensation and sensorimotor deficits), signs of hypercalcemia, functional assessment (mobility, able to dress/undress self, presence of aphasia or dysphasia), skin assessment

3. Urge incontinence: nocturia, frequency with urination

4. Stress incontinence: leakage of urine upon laughing, coughing, sneezing, lifting, or bending

5. Overflow incontinence: bladder distention, discomfort, urgency, continual dribbling and only voiding small amounts, large residual urine after voiding, fecal impaction

6. Functional incontinence: mobility, ability to perform ADLs, cognitive level, depression

D. Diagnoses

1. Altered urinary elimination related to anatomic dysfunction or obstruction, medications, or metabolic disorder

2. Urinary incontinence, urge, related to bladder irritation, sensory-motor disorder, or decreased mobility

3. Urinary incontinence, stress, related to decrease in bladder or sphincter support

4. Urinary incontinence, functional, related to cognitive dysfunction or mobility problems

5. Risk for impaired skin integrity related to urinary incontinence

6. Patient/family knowledge deficit related to etiology and management of urinary incontinence

7. Patient/family anxiety related to urinary incontinence

8. Risk for falls trying to get to the bathroom

E. Planning and intervention

1. Review medications and discontinue those that may be causing incontinence (if appropriate)

2. If appropriate, establish a regular voiding schedule (i.e., every 2 hours)

3. Alter environment to make toileting easier (i.e., move patient closer to toilet, or utilize a bedside commode, urinal, or bedpan, assuring modesty and dignity is maintained)

4. Decrease fluid intake at night, and limit intake of food/fluids containing caffeine or alcohol

5. If fecal impaction is present, disimpact and teach bowel regime to patient and family to avoid further problems

6. Consider catheterizing, either indwelling or external

7. Utilize incontinence supplies, such as pads, briefs, etc.

8. Teach patient and family hygiene and skin care measures

9. Urge incontinence: antibiotics for UTI, urinary tract analgesics such as phenazopyradine, imipramine for neurogenic bladder

10. Stress incontinence: teach pelvic floor muscle exercises and voiding schedule, pessary or penile clamp, imipramine at bedtime for anticholinergic effect

11. Overflow incontinence: discontinue anticholinergic medications, if possible; disimpact if necessary; cholinergic drug such as bethanechol; indwelling catheterization if obstruction persists

12. Functional incontinence: interventions rely on cause of incontinence; indwelling catheter may be only choice

13. Incontinence related to fistulas is treated by establishing voiding schedules, catheterization, and, if indicated, urinary diversion (if life expectancy is not short)

F.   Patient/Family Education

1.   Expected medication effects and potential side effects

2.   Demonstrate correct hygiene and skin care techniques to prevent skin breakdown

3.   Explain correct catheter care and signs of catheter malfunction

4.   Explain safety measures if altering environment for ease in toileting (i.e., have patient call for assistance, voiding schedules, assuring clear path to bathroom)

5.   Explain signs and symptoms of urinary tract infection (UTI)

G.   Evaluate

1.   Effectiveness of interventions (Are patient/family satisfied with outcome?)

2.   Skin integrity

3.   Medication effects and side effects

4.   Patient safety

H.   Revise plan: according to findings from ongoing evaluations, changes in patient/family needs

REFERENCES

1. Bergstrom, N., et al., *Pressure Ulcer Treatment: Clinical Practice Guideline. Quick Reference Guide for Clinicians, No. 15.* 1994, U.S. Department of Health and Human Services, Public Health Service, Agency for Health Care Policy and Research: Rockville, MD.

2. Barr, J.E., *Principles of wound cleansing.* Ostomy/Wound Management, 1995. **41**(Supp 7A): p. 15S-22S.

3. Dahlin, C.M. and T. Goldsmith, *Dysphagia, dry mouth, & hiccups, in Textbook of Palliative Nursing,* B.R. Ferrell and N. Coyle, Editors. 2001, Oxford University Press: New York. p. 122–138.

4. Waller, A. and N.L. Caroline, *Handbook of palliative care in cancer.* 2nd Edition ed. 2000, Boston: Butterworth-Heinemann.

5. Coda, B.A., et al., *Comparative efficacy of patient-controlled administration of morphine, hydromorphone, or sufentanil for the treatment of oral mucositis pain following bone marrow transplantation (Abstract).* Pain, 1997. **72**(3): p. Retrieved October 9, 2001 from the Ovid Bibliographic Records database.

6. Rhiner, M. and N.E. Slatkin, *Pruritis, fever, and sweats,* in *Textbook of Palliative Nursing,* B.R. Ferrell and N. Coyle, Editors. 2001, Oxford University Press: New York. p. 245–261.

7. Kuebler, K.K., N. English, and D.E. Heidrich, *Delirium, confusion, agitation, and restlessness,* in *Textbook of Palliative Nursing,* B.R. Ferrell and N. Coyle, Editors. 2001, Oxford University Press: New York. p. 290–308.

8. Taber, C.W., *Taber's cyclopedic medical dictionary.* 18th Edition ed. 1997, Philadelphia, PA: A. Davis.

9. Kuebler, K.K., *Hospice and palliative care clinical practice protocol: Terminal restlessness.* 1997, Pittsburgh, PA: Hospice and Palliative Nurses Association.

10. Collins, C.A., *Ascites.* Clinical Journal of Oncology Nursing, 2001. **5**(1): p. 43–44.

11. Kemp, C., *Terminal illness: A guide to nursing care.* 2nd Edition ed. 1999, Philadelphia, PA: Lippincott.

12. Baumrucker, S.J., *Current concepts in hospice care: Management of intestinal obstruction in hospice care.* The American Journal of Hospice and Palliative Care, 1998. **14**(4): p. 232–235.

13. Preston, F.A. and R.S. Cunningham, *Clinical guidelines for symptom management in oncology: A handbook for advanced practice nurses.* 1998, New York: Clinical Insights Press.

14. Dudgeon, D., *Dyspnea, death rattle, and cough,* in *Textbook of Palliative Nursing,* B.R. Ferrell and N. Coyle, Editors. 2001, Oxford University Press: New York. p. 164–174.

15. Grant, M., et al., *Assessment of quality of life with a single instrument.* Seminars in Oncology Nursing, 1990. **6**(4): p. 260–270.

16. Chochinov, H.M. and W. Breitbart, *Handbook of psychiatry and palliative care.* 2000, New York: Oxford University Press.

17. McCaffery, M. and C. Pasero, *Pain: Clinical Manual.* 1999, St. Louis, MO: Mosby.

18. Rousseau, P., *Nonpain symptom management in terminal care.* Clinics in Geriatric Medicine, 1996. **12**(2): p. 313–327.

19. Campbell, T. and J. Hately, *The management of nausea and vomiting in advanced cancer.* International Journal of Palliative Nursing, 2000. **6**(1): p. 18–20, 22–25.

20. Paice, J.A., *Neurological disturbances, in Textbook of Palliative Nursing,* B.R. Ferrell and N. Coyle, Editors. 2001, Oxford University Press: New York. p. 262–268.

21. Nation, R.L., A.M. Evans, and R.W. Milne, *Pharmacokinetic drug interactions with phenytoin (Part I).* Clinical Pharmacokinetics, 1997. **18**(1): p. 37–60.

GENERAL REFERENCES

Chochinov, H.M. & Breitbart, W. (2000). *Handbook of psychiatry in palliative care.* Oxford: Oxford University Press.

Head-to-toe review may find reversible cause of fatigue in cancer patient. (1995, May). *Oncology News International,* 4, 5.

Herfindal, E. T., Gourley, D. R., eds. (1996). *Textbook of therapeutics: Drug and disease management.* Baltimore: Williams & Wilkins.

Kaye, P. (1990). *Notes on symptom control in hospice and palliative care,* (Rev. 1st ed.). (USA version). Essex, CT: Hospice Education Institute.

Kuebler, K.K. (Ed.). (1996). *Hospice and palliative care clinical practice protocol: Dyspnea.* Pittsburgh, PA: Hospice and Palliative Nurses Association.

McConnell, E. A. (1994). Loosening the grip of intestinal obstructions. *Nursing, 94*(3), pp. 34–41.

Neeno, T. A. (1996). Intractable hiccups: Consider nebulized lidocaine [letter]. *Chest,* 110(4): pp. 1129–30.

Rousseau, P. (1995). Hiccups. *Southern Medical Journal,* 88(2): pp. 175–181.

Sander, R. (2000). Promoting urinary continence in residential care. *Nursing Standard,* 14(13), pp. 49–54.

Sheldon, J. (Ed.). (1999). *Hospice and palliative care clinical practice protocol: Nausea and vomiting.* Pittsburgh, PA: Hospice and Palliative Nurses Association.

Smith, S.A. (Ed.). (2001). *Hospice and palliative care clinical practice monograph: Treatment of end-stage non-cancer diagnoses.* Pittsburgh, PA: Hospice and Palliative Nurses Association.

Tips on alleviating fatigue due to cancer. (1999, November). *Primary Care and Cancer, 19,* 10.

Volker, B.G. (Ed.) (1999). *Hospice and palliative nursing practice review (3rd Ed.).* Dubuque, IA: Kendall/Hunt Publishing.

Wald, A. (1997). Fecal incontinence: Three steps to successful management. *Geriatrics,* 52(7), pp. 44–52.

Wrede-Seaman, L. (1999). *Symptom management algorithms: A handbook for palliative care.* Yakima, WA: Intellicard.

CHAPTER VI

CARE OF THE PATIENT AND FAMILY

Terry Altilio, ACSW
Judith B. Eighmy, RN, BSN, CHPN
Elayne J. Nahman, LCSW, ACSW

I. **Patient/Family Education and Advocacy—Definitions**

   A. **Education is defined as the knowledge or skill obtained or developed by a learning process; an instructive or enlightening experience**

   B. **Advocacy is defined as the act of pleading or arguing in favor of something, such as a cause, idea or policy; also see active support**

   C. **Family is defined as those individuals identified by the patient as their primary supports regardless of blood or legal ties**

   D. **Family caregivers are those unpaid individuals who provide or arrange for essential assistance to a relative or friend who is ill[1]**

II. **Caregiver Support: Access appropriate resources to meet the needs of patient and family**

   A. **Agency resources**

      1. Services of the entire Palliative Care or Hospice Interdisciplinary Team (IDT)

      2. Volunteer services

      3. Interpreters and translations of consents, educational materials, etc.

      4. Continuous home care, general inpatient or inpatient respite levels of care

      5. Placement in an appropriate setting (SNF, hospital, etc.)

      6. Support groups

B.   Patient/family resources

1.   Other family members

2.   Friends and neighbors

3.   Clergy and members of patient/family's church, synagogue, etc.

C.   Community resources—both hospice and palliative care are provided in collaboration with community resources. Hospice and palliative care nurses must be aware of existing resources and what they provide for the patient and family; examples are:

1.   Federal/state agencies, e.g., Area Agencies on Aging, Department of Health Services, Social Security Administration

2.   Charitable organizations, e.g., American Cancer Society, American Heart Association, Make-a-Wish Foundation, etc.

3.   Local churches, Temples, synagogues or other places of worship

4.   Indigent care programs through pharmaceutical companies

D.   Other information sources, e.g. Internet, public library, area medical libraries

1.   Offer respite as needed for patients and family

2.   Promote family self-care activities for hospice patients

3.   Volunteers, home health aide and homemaker services to lighten the workload

4.   Plan care to make use of other family members and friends who might provide relief for a few hours

5.   Consider another setting for care/placement for patient, i.e., skilled nursing facility

E.   Offer referral for counseling to IDT social worker or community resource counseling (Think of counseling as another form of education)

1.   Individual: a form of therapy where an individual meets regularly with a therapist; more one-on-one attention, confidentiality; example: brief psychotherapy

2.   Group: a form of therapy where a group of patients, caregivers or family members meets regularly with one another under the direction of a therapist; participants gain insight, learn stress management skills, and receive support from the therapist and others in the group; examples: support groups, bereavement groups, other specialized groups

3.   Family Meetings:

a)   Family meetings/conferences are organized around such goals as providing information, assessing practical and emotional needs, problem solving, reviewing goals of care, resolving conflict, decision making and/or validating patient and/or family efforts and stresses

b)   Such meetings are a concrete representation of health care teams interest, availability and support

c)   Decisions about who is to participate depend on the goal and purpose of the meeting; may or may not include the patient; may or may not include all team members

III. Education

A.   **Assess caregiver emotional (depression, anxiety, etc.), cognitive (fears, worries) and physical (fatigue, insomnia, symptoms, etc.) factors (strengths and limitations) to determine readiness to integrate and carry out specific tasks**

B.   **Teach primary caregivers specific techniques for patient care, e.g., medication administration, dressing changes, tube feedings**

C.   **Language and cultural variations may require adaptation of teaching tool and approaches**

    1.   Six steps to effective teaching

        a)   Step 1: State the purpose/goal/objective of the learning experience

           (1)   State purpose/goal/objective in behavioral terms

           (2)   "What and Why", creating the need to know

        b)   Step 2: Determine the needs of the learner, to match content and presentation to learner's needs

           (1)   Assess language and cultural differences, readiness and motivation of learner

           (2)   Assess literacy level, if appropriate

        c)   Step 3: Devise a plan or a method of presenting the material to the learner; include members of the Interdisciplinary Team in the planning and as instructors

           (1)   Organize yourself first

           (2)   Present things in a logical fashion

           (3)   Progress from simple to complex

           (4)   General to specific

           (5)   In chronological order

           (6)   Gather and use visual aids such as flow charts, copies of forms and samples, illustrations, key words, ideas or steps

        d)   Step 4: Provide time for the learner to clarify content

           (1)   Discuss using their own words

           (2)   Questions

           (3)   Observe

           (4)   Demonstrate

           (5)   Example

e)   Step 5: Schedule time for the learner to practice the newly acquired knowledge or skills

    (1)   Joint visits

    (2)   Patient/caregiver practice

    (3)   Observation

    (4)   Journal results

    (5)   Demonstration

    (6)   Storytelling

f)   Step 6: Schedule time for the learner's new skills to be evaluated. Involve other Interdisciplinary Team members in the evaluation process

    (1)   Joint visits

    (2)   Review

    (3)   Pictures

    (4)   Observation

    (5)   Verbal recall

    (6)   Demonstration

    (7)   "What if" sharing

2.   Utilize principles of adult learning[2]

a)   Collaborating

b)   Critically reflective thinking

c)   Learning for action

d)   Learning in a participative environment

e)   Empowering learners

f)   Dialoguing in the learning process

g)   Self-directed learning

D.   Monitor primary caregivers ability to provide care

1.   Verbalization of understanding of instructions and willingness to provide care

2.   Return demonstration of technique(s) taught

3.   Observe, support and positively reinforce actual care during patient contact, i.e., visits to home, palliative care unit, acute care setting

4.   Conduct on-going proactive assessment of caregiver physical and emotional status as over time caregiver's fatigue, mood and physical abilities change (a reality that may go unrecognized or unarticulated by the caregiver)

E. Identify and consider individualizing factors that impact ability or style of learning

1. Personal factors, e.g., patient or caregiver illiteracy, learning disabilities, impairments of vision or hearing, preferred learning style

2. Environmental challenges, e.g., noise, frequent interruptions, general chaos

3. Familial and/or cultural factors, e.g., in some cultures it is not "proper" for a daughter to provide personal care for her father

4. Language differences and communication challenges, i.e., inability to speak, read and/or write English; no available bilingual professionals, no teaching materials in preferred language

5. Emotional issues, i.e., depression, anxiety, fatigue, denial, anticipatory grieving

F. Teach about pain and symptom relief

1. See Chapters IV and V

2. See *Six Steps to Effective Teaching,* above

3. Teach complementary, non-pharmacologic modalities as well as pharmacologic methods of pain and symptom relief, e.g., cutaneous therapies (heat, cold and vibration), self-hypnosis, distraction, humor, massage, aromatherapy, etc.

G. Teach about the end-stage disease process.

1. See Chapter III

2. See *Six Steps to Effective Teaching,* above

H. Teach about the signs and symptoms of imminent death

1. See Chapter IX

2. See *Six Steps to Effective Teaching,* above

IV. Advocacy

A. Monitor needs for changes in levels of palliative/hospice care and/or Interdisciplinary Team services

1. Assess patient/family/caregiver needs at each contact

2. Encourage family/caregiver to report changes in patient status as well as changes in their own physical and emotional state when they occur

3. Encourage all team members who have patient/family contact to assess needs and report changes in patient condition and in the physical and emotional state of the caregiver and family

4. Facilitate effective communication between patient, family and care providers; sit down, minimize personal distractions, take a couple of deep breaths to focus self

5. Listen to what is being said with all your senses

6. Observe expressions, body language, etc. (Pay special attention when they do not reflect what is being said.)

7. Communicate in terms the listener understands, verbal and nonverbal

8. Be sure you understand what the speaker intended to communicate, e.g., solicit feedback

B. Assess and compensate, when possible, for barriers to communication

1. Language challenges

2. Unwillingness or inability to concentrate on what is being said

3. Lack of interest

4. Environmental challenges, e.g., noise, interruptions, physical distance

5. Physical barriers, e.g., visual or hearing impairment

C. Encourage and support patient and family in sharing their individual decision-making style regarding illness related decisions and treatment options, i.e., empower patient and family; inquire about cultural dimensions

D. In collaboration with the primary physician and other members of the IDT and with consideration of individual and cultural differences, inform patient/family of treatment options available to them

1. Assist the patient/family in clarifying their goals vs. focusing on specific treatments and/or interventions

2. Discuss with patient/family the benefits vs. the burdens of each option with consideration of both physical and psychological benefits and burdens for patient, caregiver and family members

3. Answer questions truthfully and as completely as possible

    a) Utilize available resources as needed

    b) Seek input from primary physician and other IDT members

4. Support the patient/family in the decision making process

    a) Acknowledge their right and ability to make the decision

    b) Be *non-judgmental*

    c) Assess needs of children, adolescents and extended family all along the continuum of illness to participate based on family preferences and developmental levels (See Chapter VIII, End-of-Life Care for the Dying Child and Family)

E. Make referrals for IDT consults

1. Therapy services, e.g., Physical Therapy, Speech Therapy, Occupational Therapy

2   Counseling services, e.g., spiritual, dietary, bereavement

3. Medical Social Worker for counseling, family meetings and/or counseling, group intervention, resources

4. Complementary and alternative modalities, e.g., massage therapy, music therapy

F.   Participate in advance care planning, e.g., advance directives, life support, DNR status

1.   Inform patient regarding the right of self-determination, recognizing cultural and individual preferences

a)   Be sure to identify the decision maker for the patient

b)   In some cultures the decision maker designated by legal statute may not be the decision maker designated by family or culture

2.   Assess decision-making preferences of patient and family

a)   Information and education may be helpful for some and not for others

b)   In some family settings the presence and participation of elders, clergy, healers, etc are essential

3.   Provide information and education to assist the patient/family in the decision-making process; individualize according to cultural and family belief systems that may be incongruous with advanced care planning concepts

4.   Answer questions as needed and/or refer patient/family to appropriate resources

5.   Assure patient/family that they will receive good care and treatment regardless of resuscitation status

6.   Assure patient/family of continued care in the most appropriate setting as long as they meet admission criteria and desire care by the agency or appropriate referral to another care setting

G.   Monitor care for neglect and abuse (of patient or caregiver) in collaboration with other members of the Interdisciplinary Team

1.   Physical indicators such as:

a)   Injuries not cared for properly and/or incompatible with history

b)   Evidence of inadequate care, e.g., gross pressure ulcers, soiled clothing or bed, etc.

c)   Evidence of inadequate or inappropriate administration of medication

d)   Dehydration and/or malnourishment without illness-related cause

e)   Lack of bandages on injuries or stitches when indicated, or evidence of unset bones

f)   Cuts, lacerations, puncture wounds, burns

g)   Bruises, welts, discoloration, e.g., bilateral on upper arms, morphologically similar to an object, clustered in one general area

2.   Behavioral indicators:

a)   Fear, withdrawal, helplessness, hesitation to talk openly, implausible stories, ambivalence/contradictory statements not due to mental dysfunction, resignation, non-responsiveness

b)   Presence of any of the above does not necessarily mean the individual is abused; it should alert the nurse to the possibility and to the need to continue to assess for abuse and to discuss with the other members of the Interdisciplinary Team

3. Indicators from family/caregiver:

    a) Patient/client not given the opportunity to speak for self or to be alone with nurse

    b) Family declines visits from members of the Interdisciplinary Team

    c) Absence of necessary, available assistance, attitudes of indifference or anger toward patient

    d) Family/caregiver blames patient for their illness or incapacitation

    e) Aggressive behavior toward patient or aggressive behavior toward caregiver that may emanate from patients anger, frustration at being sick, dependent or a reflection of prior abuse history

    f) Patient/family/caregiver disclosure of abuse or observation of physical, emotional abuse or neglect

4. Interventions:

    a) Confer with members of the Interdisciplinary Team especially the Social Worker; signs of neglect and abuse have multilevel etiologies such as:

        (1) Caregiver fatigue and depression

        (2) Patient anger, rage, helplessness or prior history of abuse of family

        (3) Patient's inability or unwillingness to cooperate with family/caregivers

        (4) Inadequate symptom management

    b) Report according to applicable state law

    c) If possible, inform patient/caregiver that a report is being made

V. Resource Management

A. Inform patient/family how to access hospice/palliative care services 24 hours a day and how to obtain medications, equipment, supplies

1. Patient/family provided with 24-hour telephone number to receive services from hospice or palliative care program and/or MD/HCP office

2. Patient/family instructed how and when to utilize emergency phone numbers

B. Recognize need to modify or supplement plan to accommodate psychological/socioeconomic factors

1. Collaborate with Interdisciplinary Team and refer to social worker

2. Location of care: hospital, home, board and care, long term care facility

3. Payment for services, insurance coverage, entitlements

4. Flexibility of employment; access to and use of family leave, e.g., federal Family Medical Leave Act

5. Living situation: home, apartment; resources within the home, electricity, indoor plumbing, etc.; recognize that the home has psychological significance and that changes and additions such as medical equipment to accommodate illness may create feelings of loss and require physical and psychological adaptation

6. Respect individual needs for privacy and continuity while utilizing support personnel; homemaker, attendants, volunteers, hired caregivers, and community resources

C. Assess and respond to environmental and safety factors without implying criticism

1. Risk management procedures

a) Assess safety in the home (smoke alarms, throw rugs, access to bathroom facilities, use of oxygen, etc.)

b) Assess patient and family's ability to respond to potential emergencies, including fire, power failure, weather (tornadoes, hurricanes, flood, etc.), and other natural disasters (earthquakes)

c) Advise on adaptation of the patient's home environment for safety

d) Systematic safety assessment of the environment with emphasis on prevention of falls, infection control, fire prevention, proper storage of medications

e) Instruct patient/family in procedures related to infection control, safety and emergency preparedness

f) Refer to physical or occupational therapists as needed for evaluation, adaptation of environment, equipment etc.

g) When consistent with patient/family learning style, provide printed educational materials covering appropriate topics, e.g., standard precautions, medication administration, medication actions, side effects, etc.

h) Refer to other members of the Interdisciplinary Team

i) Refer to community resources, e.g., federal/state agencies, American Cancer Society, Meals on Wheels, local churches, synagogues, etc.

j) Monitor disposal of supplies/equipment, e.g., syringes, needles

(1) Instruct patient/family on proper use, storage and disposal of supplies and equipment

(2) Arrange for delivery and pick-up of containers for disposal of biohazardous medical waste

(a) Syringes and needles—puncture proof containers

(b) Dressings—instruct family in infection control procedures; provide containers for soiled dressings

(c) Non-scheduled drugs—flushing, garbage disposal

k) Monitor Schedule II drugs, e.g., use, misuse, abuse, destroy at time of death

(1) *Use*

    (a) Follow the written policy and patient/family plan of care

    (b) Provide instruction regarding use and document same in Patient Medical Record

    (c) Suggest use of pill minders, counting and measuring devices; some agencies provide for patients

(2) *Misuse*

    (a) May occur subsequent to misunderstanding of directions

    (b) May occur subsequent to inability to tolerate patient and/or family suffering

    (c) May involve withholding of medications subsequent to unarticulated fears such as fear of effects or side effects of medication, including addiction, shortening life, sedation

(3) *Abuse*

    (a) Risk assessment—history, home environment, observation, and patterns of medication mismanagement

    (b) Recognizing signs of drug abuse

    (c) Distinguish from pseudoaddiction (relief seeking that mimics drug-seeking behavior but emanates from unrelieved pain.)

    (d) Ongoing observation and consultation with patient and family members

    (e) Interdisciplinary Team collaboration—feedback from all team members regarding their observations, input from family, and experience

    (f) Consultation with substance abuse specialist

    (g) Follow agency/institutional protocol if misuse/abuse is suspected

(4) Destroy medications at time of death:

    (a) Follow written policy

    (b) Inform family of legal requirement regarding disposition of Schedule II drugs

    (c) Be aware of personal safety concerns if family resists following stated policy

    (d) Destroy drugs in the presence of a witness

    (e) Document outcome per policy

VI. Spiritual, Psychosocial, Family and Cultural Issues

A. **Assess and respond to spiritual needs: May be raised in relationships with any IDT member who is educationally or experientially prepared and qualified to explore and share spiritual issues; consider, in consult with patient and/or family, referral to spiritual counselor, chaplain and/or community clergy**

1. Spiritual care is mandated by:

   a) Medicare hospice regulations

   b) NHPCO Standards of a Hospice Program of Care

   c) JCAHO Hospice Standards

   d) The philosophy of hospice care

   e) Palliative care standards: RWJ Last Acts Campaign

   f) World Health Organization

2. Spirituality can be described as:

   a) The search for ultimate meaning and purpose of life which may involve connection to a higher power

   b) The enhancement of a loving relationship by the individual in community

   c) The capacity to persevere with hope in the face of challenges to quality of life

   d) A way of describing the organizing center in a person's life

3. Spirituality vs. religion: Religion can be described as the formal expression on one's spirituality

4. Common concerns which can cause spiritual distress:

   a) Alienation from the religious or spiritual community

   b) Lack of access to religious or spiritual rituals or contact with faith of choice

   c) Difficulty in finding the meaning of suffering and/or approaching death; feelings such as existential distress, despair, anxiety related to the meaning of illness, suffering or death

   d) Need to reconcile with God, others, and self

   e) Spiritual beliefs opposed by family, peers, and/or health care professionals

5. Spiritual work may involve:

   a) Remembering: Taking inventory or life review

   b) Reassessing: How the patient defines him or herself in light of the life threatening illness and the life lived

   c) Reconciliation: Resolving painful breaks in relationships

   d) Reunion: Reconnecting with individuals important to the dying person

B.   Assess and respond to psychological, social and emotional status; issues are shared responsibilities and may be raised with any member of the IDT who is qualified to explore; consider referral to a Social Worker who is specifically trained in this aspect of care

1.   Psychosocial assessment of patient/family/caregiver usually includes:

   a)   Physical history, including respective perceptions of the illness and potential outcome

   b)   Goals for palliative/end-of-life care

   c)   Social history, including financial, legal and employment status

   d)   Cultural and religious considerations

   e)   Cognitive/mental status of patient and primary caregivers

   f)   Family assessment, including family structure (location and availability of caregivers and/or significant support), family dynamics, communication patterns, history of abuse or violence, substance use and abuse

   g)   Psychological evaluation including mood disorders, mental illness, suicidal ideation and previous losses

   h)   Coping skills, both past and present

   i)   Assessment of the family system for strengths and weaknesses

   j)   Caregiver availability and capability/capacity, sources of stress and vulnerability

   k)   Wills, advance directives and funeral arrangements, when culturally appropriate

   l)   Bereavement assessment (hospice and palliative care)

C.   Evaluate patient's emotional status; determine underlying cause for their behavior; collaborate with team members regarding assessment and interventions

1.   Anger or hostility

   a)   Possible causes/assessments: feelings of loneliness and helplessness, frustration, actual or anticipated loss, inability to cope, perceived threat, anxiety, abandonment, actual or perceived loss of control and autonomy

   b)   Management options: encourage verbalization and exploration of reasons for the anger, reassure family and other caregivers that anger may be frequently misplaced and in that setting ought not to be taken personally, assist patient to examine and improve self-concept, assist patient to identify opportunities for increased and enhanced feelings of control

   c)   Anxiety

   d)   Possible causes/assessments: difficult to assess; be sure symptom management is optimized, evaluate medication effects, requires careful team assessment and management. Etiology may include physical factors, medications, psychological/existential distress. Symptoms may include palpitations, shortness of breath, diaphoresis, increased fear, helplessness and loss of control. May be related to medical problems, pain medications, abnormal mental states, withdrawal phenomenon

e) Management options: treat underlying cause, if appropriate; reassurance for patient and family, use of anxiolytic medications as appropriate, use of other therapies such as relaxation, guided imagery, cognitive interventions, supportive counseling. Provide continuity, consistency and predictability in environment and care giving

2. Denial

    a) Possible causes/assessments: inability to cope with bad news, disbelief and fear; differentiate denial from avoidance

        (1) Denial is an unconscious process designed to protect against an overwhelming reality

        (2) Avoidance is a conscious process that protects patients from bringing distressing aspects of their reality to the forefront

    b) Management options: allow denial as a coping mechanism (once it is known information was indeed given), continue to answer questions honestly (don't encourage the denial), avoid confrontation, avoid giving information not requested

3. Depression (See Table: *Key Differences Between Grieving and Depression*)

    a) Possible causes/assessments: difficult to assess since the usual indicators of depression, including disturbed sleep, anorexia, weariness, constipation, reduced libido, emotional lability, are also present subsequent to illness and/or treatments; requires careful team assessment and management with particular attention to emotional factors such as hopelessness, helplessness, low self esteem, guilt

    b) Management options: treat underlying cause, if appropriate; control of symptoms, assuring patients will remain in control of their care; antidepressant medications when appropriate, referral for professional counseling, cognitive behavioral interventions

4. Fear

    a) Possible causes/assessments: potential pain, potential abandonment, financial crisis, potential dependency, potential death, spiritual concerns

    b) Management options: encourage verbalization, patient teaching if operating under wrong information, accept fears as real (don't minimize), social work or spiritual counselor referral if appropriate

5. Grief

    a) Possible causes/assessments: perceived loss of self, meaning, or other valued entities

    b) Management options: encourage expressions of grief, permit crying, use written and verbal information about the normalcy of grief reactions, be a good listener, encourage person to tell their story

6. Guilt

    a) Possible causes/assessments: unresolved issues with God or others, feelings of failure, ambivalence, poor relationships, inappropriate expectations, dependence

    b) Management options: normalize feelings when appropriate; encourage ventilation, completion of unfinished business, referral to social work and/or spiritual counselor if appropriate

7. Impaired communication

   a) Possible causes/assessments: head and neck cancer, laryngectomy, depression, paralysis, aphasia, emotional angst

   b) Management options vary with the cause:

      (1) If the cause has an emotional basis, use therapeutic silence (merely being present without being uncomfortable), ask open-ended questions, provide adequate response time, gain trust by good physical care and sharing information, convey empathy

      (2) If the cause is physical, teach communication skills and provide support, devise non-verbal response plan such as hand squeeze, nod or eye blink when appropriate, referral to Speech-Language Pathologist as appropriate, use of communication devices, ask questions that can be answered by single words

8. Loss of hope or meaning

   a) Possible causes/assessments: grief, overwhelming pain or disability, spiritual distress, emotional overload, fear of death, depression

   b) Management options:

      (1) Effective symptom management to ensure that any physical causes are addressed

      (2) Acknowledge feelings; social work/spiritual counselor, if appropriate; evaluate for depression/consider antidepressants

      (3) Guide patient to identify priorities and achievable goals and to broaden the scope of hope and hope-related activities beyond cure of illness

      (4) Encourage life review; allow patient to maintain control by offering options and choices

9. Near death awareness

   a) Possible causes/assessments: dreams or visions of deceased people, God, or heaven; acceptance of immortality, talk about a trip or a journey, fear of being alone; assess the special awareness, needs, and communications of the dying

   b) Management options: encourage verbalization without judgment or interpretation, encourage family to be present and share important messages with patient, listen for meaning or meaningful experiences, distinguish between "confusion" and symbolic communication (i.e., "going home" may not refer to a physical place but may mean heaven or another concept of an afterlife)

10. Sleep disturbances

    a) Possible causes/assessments: can be multivariate, often with a physical and emotional basis; ascertain if alcohol, caffeine, theophylline or theobromine-containing foods/fluids are a contributing factor; a complete symptom assessment is essential!

b)   Management options: treat underlying cause, if appropriate: explore meaning for the patient and family; be sure all symptoms are optimally controlled; a trial with a variety of sedative and hypnotic drugs may be useful, teach sleep hygiene; replicate previous sleep rituals; consider non-pharmacological interventions such as music therapy, guided imagery, warm milk, suggest limiting intake of alcohol, caffeine, theophylline and theobromine containing foods/fluids especially at night

11.   Spiritual distress or unresolved spiritual issues

a)   Possible causes/assessments: guilt, regrets, lack of meaning, poor relationships, fear of unknown; assess value of rituals to patient

b)   Management options: acknowledge spiritual pain, encourage verbalization, use a family genogram to elicit values, relationships, fears, hopes and unfinished business; provide requested prayers, readings, hymns, or spiritual counselors; respect individual belief systems, explore issues related to forgiveness for possible resolution

12.   Suicidal or homicidal ideation

a)   Possible causes/assessments: despair, clinical depression, need for control hopelessness, anger, unrelieved pain, delirium; evaluate reasons and degree of intent (i.e., is there a plan?), evaluate elements of patient's suffering, feelings of being a burden

b)   Management options: Consult agency policies & procedures, consult with team, provide adequate pain and symptom management, plan interventions to ameliorate causes of suffering, increase opportunities for control, provide care that supports dignity, consider antidepressants, involve close family member or friend to support patient, encourage patient to talk about suicidal or homicidal thoughts, formulate a "contract" with patient, psychiatric or crisis center referral if appropriate

13.   Unresolved interpersonal matters

a)   Possible causes/assessments: poor coping, distance, busyness, addictions, knowledge deficit, abuse, psychiatric or personality disorders

b)   Management options: encourage patient to prioritize concerns, offer pertinent information if desired, encourage family involvement, use family tree to elicit information, ascertain degree of help patient desires, referral to professional counseling

D.   Assess and respond to family systems and dynamics, both palliative care services and hospice include the patient and family as the unit of care

1.   The family as a system

a)   A complex entity comprised of interrelated and interacting individuals functioning within a socio-economic, political, environment as well as a health care setting

b)   Primary object of system is to maintain equilibrium in environment, which facilitates individual and family development

c)   System seeks to maintain equilibrium through dynamic process of homeostasis

2. Terms and definitions

a) *Boundary*—A term used in family therapy to describe emotional barriers that protect and enhance the integrity of individuals, subsystems and families

b) *Enmeshment*—A term for the loss of autonomy due to a blurring of psychological boundaries

c) *Triangulation*—Detouring conflict between two people by involving a third person, stabilizing the relationship between the original pair

d) *Disengaged*—Opposite of enmeshed. Family members pay no attention to or disregard one another

e) *Differentiation*—Psychological separation of intellect and emotions, and independence of self from others

f) *Homeostasis*—A balanced steady state of equilibrium

g) *Family homeostasis*—Tendency of families to resist change in order to maintain a steady state. The ability to adapt over time to changes

h) *Reframing*—Re-labeling a family's perception or description of behavior or an experience to make it more amenable to change or less threatening

i) *Systems, closed*—A functionally related group of elements regarded as forming a collective entity that does not interact with the surrounding environment

j) *Systems, open*—A set of interrelated elements that exchange energy and material with the surrounding environment

k) *Genogram*—A schematic diagram of the family system, using geometrical shapes to represent individuals and their position within the family

3. Additional family assessment parameters

a) Adaptation to chronic, life-threatening illness

b) Family develops response patterns to crisis, which is often repeated

c) Reaction to illness influenced by family's historical responses, reaction to stress, role flexibility, decision making process, their communication, past and present with the health care team, gender, socio-economic variables and sexual orientation

d) Stressors on the family system

(1) Horizontal stressors:

(a) Family's experience with normal strains of development and life cycle transitions (marriage, birth, and death)

(b) Environmental stressors may include financial stresses, ongoing illness-related demands, substance abuse or other unexpected events

(c) Interview questions should address the impact of the illness on the completion of the family's developmental tasks, external events and coping strategies

(2) Vertical stressors:

(a) Behavioral, relational and emotional and belief patterns inherited from past generations

(b) Interview questions should address historical coping styles and family history of loss, family values, fractured relationships and spirituality

E. Assess and respond to cultural and ethnic variations

1. Modify the plan of care to accommodate cultural and ethnic diversity

a) Be open to varying degrees of cultural and individual differences that require modification of interventions and plan of care

b) Ask patients and families about their cultural beliefs, values and practices. The culture of the patient and family may be different from the culture of the health care professionals, creating challenges to communication and understanding. Keep in mind:

(1) Stereotyping—do not assume that all people from a particular country, region, or nationality hold identical beliefs and practices

(2) Assimilation—A person from another culture or ethnic group who has been in the United States for several generations may no longer follow the customs of their native heritage or speak the language

(3) At times of crises the generational differences may cause conflicts or create circumstances where the assimilated generations return to the rituals and comfort of earlier beliefs

2. Multi-culturalism—ethnic background includes many different nationalities

3. It is important to explore the following areas, which may be impacted by cultural and religious facets

a) Time orientation i.e., emphasis on past versus present versus future

b) Appropriate clothing, food preferences, traditional and folk remedies

c) Issues related to gender, privacy, touch, eye contact and personal space

d) Decision-making style: self determination/autonomy versus family, community decision making style

e) Communication, truth-telling, direct, open, non-verbal, use of silence

f) Taboos, rituals, healing practices

g) What is acceptable (dying at home, discontinuing treatments, medically provided nutrition/hydration, organ donation, etc.)

h) Customs and belief systems related to transitions (reincarnation, after-life, etc.)

i) Specific practices related to illness, pain, treatments, suffering and end-of-life, relationship to health care providers

j) Other considerations: What are the norms? Prohibitions?

k) Language differences require use of translators other than family members who translate information through the filter of their own suffering, cognitive and emotional response to the illness

4. Basic beliefs regarding death and dying and afterlife for some of the major subcultures and religions:

    a) African-American:

        (1) Cannot make a definitive statement about the dying and mourning process because of the diversity that exists across such a wide and varied community including religious dominations, geographical regions, educational backgrounds, and the economic levels of the families and communities involved

        (2) Some aspects that have been virtually universal in recent times are that funerals tend to be highly involved ceremonies with defined rituals and all efforts will be made by family, friends and even acquaintances of the deceased to attend

    b) Latino/Hispanic: Largest and youngest ethnic minority in U.S.

        (1) Many subcultures within this population with diverse cultural variations (i.e. Mexico, Central America, the Caribbean, Venezuela, etc.)

        (2) Catholicism is the predominant religion but many depend on folk healers or spiritualists for their ailments

        (3) Death is viewed as a direct result of life, one naturally follows the other

        (4) There is an acceptance of death due to past experience with death, poverty, religion, and culture; family and family life is important, especially surrounding death and funerals; open expression of grief particularly among the women

    c) Hmong: several subgroups (from China, Vietnam, Laos, Thailand, Burma)

        (1) Death and the afterlife are closely intertwined with the traditional Hmong religion which is mixture of ancestor worship and animism

        (2) The spiritual world co-exists with the physical world and spirits can influence human life

        (3) Believes that each person has several souls and that a person has a certain allotted time on earth

        (4) Healing ceremonies are thought to appease the spirits

        (5) Proper burial and worship of the dead (and other ancestors) directly affect the health, safety and prosperity of the family so considerable effort is placed on funeral process; specific rituals and ceremonies are individualized for each family line; burial always happens in the afternoon

    d) Native Americans: Over 350 distinct tribes in U.S. with much variation in terms of cultural practices

        (1) Focus of identity is on tribe rather than ancestry and each tribe has its own belief system

        (2) Universal to most tribes is the belief that "spirits" are attached to living things; acceptance of an Indian healer (Shaman); family is usually a large extended unit, often as many as a hundred or more

(3) Other considerations include: family may not want patient to die at home, but to allow a family member to die alone is also not appropriate; material possessions often are dispersed before or after death to friends and family members; bereavement follow-up may not be appropriate as some tribes have a taboo against speaking of the dead

e) Judaism (Orthodox, Conservative and Reformed):

(1) Belief in the sacredness of life and one, indivisible God

(2) Funeral has two common themes: honor the dead and comfort the mourners; body must not be left unattended until burial which should take place as soon as possible (preferably within 24 hours)

(3) Autopsies and cremation are opposed

(4) Deceased is dressed in a white shroud and buried in plain pine box

(5) A 7-day mourning period (Shiva) follows for the immediate next of kin

(6) Due to acculturation to American society, may be some variations in funeral and grief traditions

f) Buddhist (several different sects):

(1) Everything is done to ensure a calm and peaceful environment for the person who is dying

(2) View death as an opportunity for improvement in the next life, so the state of the mind at the time of death is extremely important; emphasis on mind being clear so there is general reluctance to use medications that sedate or cloud the mind

(3) After death, body should be covered and not touched or moved; when possible, there should be a 3-day wait before embalming or cremating body

(4) Funeral is planned by family members; family wears traditional white clothing and openly show grief

g) Asian (encompasses several countries and religions, i.e. East Indian, Chinese, Filipino, Japanese, Laotians, Cambodians, Korean, Vietnamese): due to large, diverse population, it is difficult to give specifics but some general beliefs:

(1) Traditional strong family and extended family with male dominance

(2) Herbal medicine plays an important role

(3) Direct eye contact considered impolite; indirect communication patterns

(4) The number or character "4" should be avoided (symbolizes death)

(5) Funeral and burial customs vary greatly depending on culture, religion and generation involved

F. **Support patient/family to facilitate anticipatory grieving and to promote healthy grieving following the death of the patient**

1. Ensure adequate symptom management along the continuum of illness; this has the potential to positively impact grief of surviving family members

2. Support and encourage life review with and without family/significant others

3. Present topics for discussion: childhood events, holidays and special celebrations

4. Use audio/visual tools: photographs, memorabilia, music

5. Encourage patient and/or family reminiscences, work, losses, accomplishment, disappointments, early years, etc.

G. **Provide death vigil support and expertise, as the manner of death will impact the surviving family members' perceptions and the way in which the death is integrated into the family history**

1. Management of acute physical symptoms

2. Provide support for the family and dignity for the patient

H. **Visit at time of death whether at home, in hospital or long term care facility**

1. The task and focus will be determined by the place of death, and may include facilitating pronouncement, notification and transportation

2. Attendance at death provides support for patient and family

I. **Facilitate transition into bereavement services**

1. Provide emotional support to family during and at the time of death

2. Acknowledge reactions to grief

3. Notify bereavement coordinator or designee according to agency policy for follow-up

4. Counsel or provide emotional support regarding grief and loss for adults. Ten counseling principles[3]

   a) Help the survivor actualize the loss

   b) Help the survivor to identify and express feelings

   c) Assist living without the deceased

   d) Facilitate emotional location of the deceased

   e) Provide time to grieve

   f) Interpret "normal" grief behavior

   g) Allow for individual differences

   h) Provide continuing support

   i) Examine defenses and coping styles

   j) Refer those who need further intervention to appropriate professionals/resources

5.   Participate in formal closure activity, e.g., visit, call, sympathy card

    a)   Condolence call made by RN Case Manager and/or other Interdisciplinary Team members. (This may be a designated task.)

    b)   Participate in signing of sympathy card for family

    c)   Attend patient's funeral/memorial service, if appropriate, as per policy and for personal/professional relationship with family

    d)   Closure visit with survivors. Arrange visit or phone call to assess family coping and to begin process of closure

    e)   Seek and accept or create individual ritual or process for integrating loss including support of the IDT for own grief

    f)   Attend Program's memorial services

VII. Grief and Loss

A.   Theory and concepts of grief and loss

1.   Definitions of key concepts:

    a)   Bereavement *is the event:* the death, the divorce, the job loss, the loss of money, the loss of self-esteem, home, the move to a new locality, of children leaving home

    b)   Grief *is the emotional feeling:* anger, frustration, loneliness, sadness, guilt, regret, related to the *perception* of the loss

    c)   Mourning *is the process of resolving the grief:* mourning has a beginning, the loss; and it can have an ending, the resolution

    d)   Grief Counseling: helping people facilitate uncomplicated or normal grief to a healthy completion of the task of grieving

    e)   Grief Therapy: specialized techniques which are used to help people with abnormal or complicated grief reactions

2.   "Normal" grief (refer also to charts following): Four tasks of Grief[3]

    a)   To accept the reality of the loss

    b)   To experience the pain of grief

    c)   To adjust to an environment in which the deceased is missing

    d)   To withdraw emotional energy and reinvest it in another relationship

3.   Abnormal, complicated or pathological grief (refer to charts following)

    a)   Absent grief: feelings of mourning totally absent

    b)   Inhibited grief: a lasting inhibition of many manifestations of normal grief; other symptoms such as somatic complaints are in their place

    c)   Delayed grief: may be delayed many years; losses precipitated by lack of support, or too little time to grieve or multiple losses; full grief reaction may occur years later initiated by another loss or event

d) Conflicted grief: ambivalent relationship with deceased is often antecedent; frequently a distortion of the elements of normal grief, i.e., an exaggeration of one aspect and suppression of another (anger and guilt)

e) Chronic grief: a continuous expression of the intense grief usually associated with the early stages of a loss; attributed to a high degree of insecurity of the bereaved, who was highly dependent on the deceased; intense mourning is a way to keep the person "alive".

f) Unanticipated grief: occurs after a sudden, extremely disruptive loss; mourners unable to grasp the full implications of the loss and may be so overwhelmed that functioning is significantly impaired

g) Abbreviated grief: often mistaken for unresolved grief, but may be a short-lived normal form; occurs following periods of extended anticipatory grief, or in situations of minimal attachment to deceased

Key Differences Between Normal and Pathological Grief

Time since loss	Most intense reactions are seen prior to six months.	Intense reactions last longer than six months with little sign of resolution or relief.
Reality testing of the loss	Holding on strategies: wants to believe the loss can be restored but know it cannot. Reality testing (after initial phase of shock) is intact.	Continues to operate as if loss was still there. Chronic, continuing hope for return of lost person or object. Refusal to actively reality test.
Preoccupation	Variable: can be intensely focused on loss or able to function. Acute awareness of what happened at time of loss: emotionally, physically, and cognitively.	Active: seeking reunion with lost object or person or clear ongoing disruption and dysfunction in daily routine; acute awareness of what happened at the time of the loss is usually cognitive only.
Dreams/imagery	Manifest content of dreams is variable but contains recognition of the absence of what has been lost.	Manifest content focused on attempts to save or destroy what (whom) was lost.
Approach/avoidance behaviors	Ambivalent about dealing with loss but willing to do so.	Avoids situations that would remind bereaved of the loss.
Intellectual/emotional integration	Intellectual and emotional awareness of loss.	Intellectual awareness only or emotional awareness without linking to intellectual awareness.

Reprinted with permission of John M. Schneider

Comparison of Grief with Depression

Issue	Grieving	Depression
Is there a loss?	Yes	Maybe/maybe not
What do they think about?	At times, they may be obsessed with the loss. At other times, they can think of other things.	Often obsessed with themselves and how this loss is unfair or a punishment.
What are their dreams & fantasies?	Vivid, clear dreams, sometimes of the loss, which can sometimes be comforting.	Flashbacks, nightmares, same disturbing dreams over and over
What is the physical effect?	Gains or loses some weight; Exercises a lot or stops entirely. Has trouble getting to sleep. Feels tired a lot.	Weight change is extreme. Exercise is also at extremes. Has trouble getting up; awakens with disturbing dreams. Always restless or always sleeping or tired.
What is the spiritual effect?	A connection is felt to something beyond the self, e.g., a belief in God and that this is happening for a reason. Able to challenge, revise, or maintain previously held beliefs.	Especially a year or more past a loss, a persistent failure to find meaning and a continued focus on "why me," on the unfairness & meaninglessness of the loss. Resists any "pat" answers when they question beliefs. Tends to discard previously held beliefs.
How do they feel?	Moody: Shifts in mood from anger to sadness to more positive feelings in the same day.	Can be hard to "read" emotionally, or they can be at an extreme, either crying all the time or not at all, angry all the time or not at all. Rarely feels "good."
How do they respond to others?	Generally respond to warmth, pressure, and reassurance. They appreciate being left alone but not ignored.	Either can't stand people at all or can't be without them. They respond to promises and urging or they remain unresponsive. Often feels abandoned and unloved when alone.
What happens to having pleasurable experiences?	As long as the pleasure isn't something that only came from the loss (e.g. sex after losing partner), it can be okay.	Either extreme they eat, drink, and are merry or they experience no pleasure at all.
How do they attach and relate to others?	Likes to have close friends or someone who will listen to their story. Misses being loved or able to love others.	Feels unloved and incapable of loving and often goes about proving it!

©2001 John Schneider reprinted with permission   * not to be distributed without permission

REFERENCES

1. Levine, C., *The many worlds of family caregivers, in Always on Call: When Illness Turns Families into Caregivers*, C. Levine, Editor. 2000, United Hospital Fund: New York. p. 1–17.

2. Leonard, D.J., *Workplace education: Adult education in a hospital nursing staff development department*. Journal of Nursing Staff Development, 1993. **9**: p. 68–73.

3. Worden, J.W., *Grief counseling and grief therapy*. 2nd Edition ed. 1991, New York: Springer.

GENERAL REFERENCES

Abrahm, J.L. (2000). *A physician's guide to pain and symptom management in cancer patients*. Baltimore, MD:Johns Hopkins University Press.

Aspen Reference Group. (1996) *Palliative care patient and family counseling manual*. Gaithersburg, MD: Aspen Publishers

Beresford, L. (1997). The updated book on prayer: Spiritual care strives to hold its place on the hospice team. *Hospice,* 8(1), 22–26.

California Association for Health Services at Home, Hospice Section Steering Committee. (1995) *Diversity and Hospice Care.*

Carson, V.B. (Ed.). (1989). *Spiritual dimensions of nursing practice*. Philadelphia: W.B. Saunders.

Case, B. (1996). Breathing AIR into adult learning. *The Journal of Continuing Education in Nursing*, 27(4), 148–158

Derrickson, B.S. (1996). The spiritual work of the dying: A framework & case studies. *The Hospice Journal, 11*(2), 11–30.

Doka, K.J. and J.D. Davison, Eds. (1998) L*iving With grief: Who we are; How we grieve*. Washington, D.C.: Hospice Foundation of America.

Dowd, S.B., et. al. (1998) "Death, dying and grief in a transcultural context: Application of the Giger and Davidhizar Assessment Model." *The Hospice Journal*. 13(4)

Geissler, E.M. (1994). *Pocket guide: Cultural assessment*. St. Louis: C.V. Mosby

Hay, M., (1996). Spiritual caregiver: The challenge of chaplaincy. *The Hospice Professional, Autumn,* 14–15.

Irish, D.P., Lundquist, K.F., & Nelson, V.J. (Eds.). (1993). *Ethnic variations in dying, death, and grief*. Washington, DC: Taylor & Francis.

Johnson, C. and McGee, M. (Eds.). (1998). *How different religions view death and afterlife,* (2nd ed.). Philadelphia: The Charles Press.

Johnson-Taylor, E., Amenta, M. & Highfield, M. (1995). Spiritual care practices of oncology nurses. *Oncology Nursing Forum*. 22(1), 31–39.

Johnson-Taylor, E., Highfield, M., & Amenta, M.(1994). Attitudes and beliefs regarding spiritual care: A survey of cancer nurses. *Cancer Nursing*. 17(6), 479–487.

Larson, D. (1993). *The helper's journey: Working with people facing grief, loss, and life-threatening illness*. Champaign, IL: Research Press.

Lemon, M., Michael, R., & Dickinson, E. (1990). *Understanding dying, death, and bereavement.* Chicago, IL: Holt, Rinehart & Winston.

Lipson, J.G., Dibble, S.L. and Minarik, P.A. (Eds.). (1996). *Culture and nursing care: A pocket guide.* San Francisco: UCSF Nursing Press.

McCaffery, M. and C. Pasero. (1999). *Pain clinical manual,* 2nd Edition. St. Louis: Mosby, Inc.

Rando, T.A. (1984). *Grief, dying and death: Clinical interventions for caregivers.* Champaign, IL: Research Press.

Rando, T. (1988). *How to go on living when someone you love dies.* Des Plains, IA: Bantam Books.

Rosen, E. (1990). *Families facing death: Family dynamics of terminal illness.* New York: Lexington Books (Simon & Schuster).

Schneider, J.M. (1994) *Finding my way: Healing and transformation through loss and grief.* Colfax, WI: Seasons Press.

Stepnick, A. & Perry, T. (1992). Preventing spiritual distress in the dying client. *Journal of Psychosocial Nursing,* 30(1), 17–24

Vachon, M.L. (1987). *Occupational stress in the care of the critically ill, the dying and the bereaved.* Philadelphia: Hemisphere Publishing.

Vachon, M.L. (1993) Emotional problems in palliative medicine: patient, family and professional. In D. Doyle, WC Hanks & N McDonald (Eds). *Oxford book of palliative medicine.* Oxford: Oxford University Press.

Walsh, D. (1990). Continuing care in a medical center: the Cleveland Clinic Foundation Palliative Care Service. *Journal of Pain and Symptom Management,* 5, 273–278.

Wholihan, D. (1992, Mar/Apr). The value of reminiscence in hospice care. *The American Journal of Hospice and Palliative Care* . pp. 33–35.

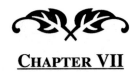

CHAPTER VII

THE DYING PATIENT AND FAMILY IN TRADITIONAL CARE SETTINGS

Marianne LaPorte Matzo, Ph.D., RN, CS
Joanne E. Sheldon, RN, MEd, CHPN, CIC

I. **The Challenge for Nurses to Provide Quality End of Life Care**

    A. **There are opportunities for nursing leadership in providing quality end-of-life care in settings other than the traditional "hospice environment"**

    B. **Attention to the unique needs of patients and families at this time reflects a commitment to nursing excellence**

    C. **Mandates to integrate palliative care principles across illness trajectories and care settings stem from the increased awareness of inadequacies of care of the dying patients and their families**

        1. As the population ages, and the incidence of chronic, progressive illness continues to increase there will be increased demands from patients and families as well as health care providers to have established standards of care for the dying and their families

        2. To respond to the demands, the nursing profession must ensure that core competencies in EOL care serve as a foundation to guide professional nurses in expert care of the dying

    D. **Nursing is in the unique position to institute change/improvement within the system since the nurse is the conduit for assessing the needs of the patient and implementing the goals of a team care plan/treatment**

    E. **The following content is applicable when providing end-of-life nursing care in any setting**

II.   The Need for Improved Care at the End of Life (EOL)

A.   Death and dying in America: Changes over the last century

1.   Late 1800s:

    a)   Health care professionals had little to offer the sick beyond the easing of symptoms associated with disease

    b)   Most deaths occurred at home with extended family members caring for the dying person[1,2]

    c)   Most died within days of onset of illness

2.   Early to middle 1900s (growth of science and industry brought about broad, sweeping changes)

    a)   Improvements in living and working conditions, sanitation, and an emphasis on disease prevention

    b)   Life-saving and life-prolonging treatments such as antibiotics, cardiopulmonary resuscitation, and advances in anesthesia[3]

    c)   The focus of health care shifted from easing suffering to curing disease

    d)   Society's expectations changed regarding treatments and interventions for curable as well as incurable illnesses[4]

        (1)   Patients whose disease failed to respond to treatments were given less priority

        (2)   Death itself became equated with medical failure[2]

3.   Demographics and social trends

    a)   Decreased age-adjusted death rate

    b)   Increased life expectancy; as death rates declined, life expectancy rose sharply, and has been primarily linked to the reduction in infant and child mortality[1]

    c)   Racial and ethnic differences:

        (1)   Significant variations exist among racial, ethnic, age, sex, and economic status sub-groups

        (2)   Variations often highlight serious gaps in access to health care and adequate EOL care

        (3)   In most cases, socially disadvantaged individuals experience higher mortality rates and death at a younger age[1,5,6]

    d)   Aging of the population

        (1)   Those > 65 years represent a progressively larger number and proportion of the population due to changing mortality patterns

        (2)   By the year 2030, as the baby boom generation reaches the age of 65, there will be approximately 70 million older persons, more than double the number in 1997[7]

4. Site of death

    a) Institutions have replaced the home as the most common place where death occurs

    b) Care is more likely to be given by strangers/health care professionals than family members[1]

5. Disease and dying trajectories illustrate differences in the dying experience by examining the duration of the dying process and the course of the disease or injury [3, 8, 1]

    a) Sudden, unexpected death

    b) Steady decline, short terminal phase

    c) Slow decline, periodic crises, and death

6. Impact

    a) Americans are living longer

    b) The period of time of living with progressive and eventually fatal illness is generally prolonged and often marked by functional dependency on others

    c) There is a trend toward the separation of family members by great distances

    d) An individual may not experience the death of a significant other until well into his/her adult years

        (1) Isolation from the death experience increases discomfort with death and the dying process

        (2) These individuals are at risk of an increased, profound emotional response to the death of a relative, friend, or other significant person[1, 3, 9]

    e) Scientific and technological advances have led to the medicalization of care at the end of life; efforts toward cure and eliminating physiological dysfunction often overshadow the obligation to provide appropriate treatment and compassionate care[10]

    f) The shift to a curative focus may actually bring about hope for cure of disease; the fact that some diseases have been cured leads to therapeutic optimism

    g) Health professionals have become increasingly uncomfortable in addressing end of life concerns with patients and families

7. SUPPORT Study

    a) The Study to Understand Prognosis and Preferences for Outcomes and Risks of Treatment

    b) Substantial shortcomings exist in care for seriously ill, hospitalized adults

    c) To improve the experience of seriously ill and dying patients, greater individual and societal commitment and more proactive and forceful measures may be needed[11]

B.   Disparity between the way people die, and the way they want to die

1.   Patient/family perspective

a)   Most adults prefer to be cared for at home if terminally ill and the majority would be interested in a comprehensive program of EOL care, such as hospice

b)   The majority of adults (62% of those surveyed) believe it would take a year or more to adjust to the death of a loved one[12]

c)   The two greatest fears associated with death are being a burden to family and being in pain[12]

d)   Many have come to fear the prospect of prolonged death characterized by over-treatment and the use of life-sustaining technology and invasive, debilitating treatments

e)   Patients and families worry that when "nothing more can be done", their health care providers will abandon them

f)   Past experiences with the death of others may influence fears about unrelieved symptoms and increased dependence on others

g)   Families may be uncertain about how to provide physical care and adjust to role changes[13]

h)   Many families drain life savings in order to cover costs of care for terminally ill family members[14]

2.   Barriers to quality care at the end of life

a)   The realities of life-limiting diseases

(1)   Failure to acknowledge the limits of medicine may lead to futile care

(2)   Inappropriate use of aggressive curative treatments can prolong the dying process and contribute to physical and emotional distress

b)   Lack of adequate training of professionals

(1)   Professionals often receive little training regarding the safe and effective means of controlling pain and other symptoms, as well as strategies to address the physical, psychological, social and spiritual aspects of care

(2)   Many health professionals are uncomfortable communicating bad news and prognosis

(3)   Nurses cannot practice what they do not know; educational efforts must incorporate the preparation of students for a professional role that includes providing quality nursing care to those approaching death[15]

c)   Delayed access to hospice and palliative care services

(1)   Services not well understood

(2)   Lack of understanding of what comprehensive EOL programs offer leads to confusion over when it is appropriate to consult or transfer care to these services

(3)   More timely referrals are necessary in order for patients and families to reap the full benefit of hospice and palliative care services

(4) Surveys indicate that patients prefer to die at home, yet only 29 percent of terminally ill patients enroll in hospice programs[1, 16]; the numbers are higher (approximately 50%) for cancer patients[17]

d) Rules and regulations

(1) Institutional regulations that impede good EOL care include restrictive visiting hours and inadequate policies for pain and symptom management

(2) Regulation of controlled substances has led to fear of prosecution for prescribing and administering medications to relieve pain and other symptoms

(3) Issues regarding access to care, insurance coverage, and the potential need to hire a caregiver from outside the family contribute to financial barriers to care

C. Costs of end of life care

1. Managed care

   a) Today patients admitted to hospitals are more critically ill, length of stay has decreased, and there is an increase in the use of ambulatory services

      (1) Patients discharged to the home and long-term care facilities are more seriously ill

      (2) There is a trend towards increased utilization of home care services[18]

   b) The health care system is straining under the effects of rapid change, making the implementation of comprehensive EOL care more difficult

   c) Certain managed care plan restrictions particularly affect people with advanced illness[1] such as:

      (1) Limiting the scope of benefits to reduce costs

      (2) Financial incentives for practitioners and providers to provide less care

      (3) Patient services that require pre-authorization

      (4) Coverage for services provided only by designated physicians and health care providers

2. Expenses for care at the end of life

   a) Spending for end of life care in a particular year may not reflect the cumulative cost of care for an illness with a long disease/dying trajectory compared with costs of intensive treatment for an illness with a short trajectory

   b) Increased costs and health care spending for end of life care are influenced by factors such as the population growth, general inflation in the economy, and medical inflation[1]

   c) Evaluation of outcomes and costs of care is necessary to validate palliative care services; continued development and utilization of outcome indicators should provide an objective evaluation of care and the development of standards to guide program development[19]

3. Payment for care at the end of life

   a) Public funding:

   (1) Efforts to control costs and reduce spending are placing increased pressure on Medicare, Medicaid and Social Security programs[1]

   (2) Medicare: covers 83% of those who die each year who are age 65 or older; and younger persons with disabilities and certain illnesses

   (3) Medicaid pays for a smaller portion of health care costs and larger portion of long-term care

   b) Other

   (1) Private insurance;

   (2) Programs servicing veterans

   (3) Out of pocket payments by patient/family

D.) Access to end of life care

   1.) Current trends that limit access include:

   a) Restrictive rules regarding eligibility

   b) The tendency to discourage new enrollment or to continue enrollment of sicker individuals in certain health plans

   c) Poor access for populations at risk: the elderly, pediatric patients, the homeless, and the uninsured

   d) Delayed referral to hospice and palliative services

   e) Reluctance of physician to refer—not wanting to look like this is "giving up on the patient"

   f) Family may not request referral or may be reluctant to accept referral when offered

   g) Cultural barriers

E. Resource allocation for end of life care

   1. Determining the benefit of treatments or therapies:

   a) Does a treatment or therapy match the patient/family goals for care?

   b) Do the benefits out-weigh the risks?

   2. Allocation questions are shadowed by questions of cost; everything that can be done to ensure comfort and quality life closure should be pursued

   3. Nurses must be conscious of financial costs as well as the burden of treatments and therapies on the patient/family

F. **Optimum use of community resources for end of life care**

    1.   Interdisciplinary teamwork extends to community resources

    2.   Early access of needed resources can significantly decrease stressors and the perception of burden especially for patients/families that do not have extended family to assist the primary caregiver

G. **Denial of death**

    1.   Reluctance to take away "hope" may delay accessing needed services, and may be one of the biggest barriers[8]

    2.   Poor communication about patient and family preferences can impede timely referrals to comprehensive end-of-life services

H. **Patient/family perspective of end of life care**

    1.   Caring for a dying patient can exhaust a family's financial resources[1] because of missed work and out of pocket medical costs

    2.   An increasing amount of payment for care has shifted to the patient/family; for persons on limited budgets this may mean they are not able to stay at home because the hiring of assistive personnel is often too costly[14]

    3.   The inability to access services that allow patients to remain at home which forces them, instead, to turn to nursing homes or other institutional care that actually increases costs of care covered by private and public sources[20]

I. **Outcomes of end of life care**

    1.   American society does not view any death (even an expected one) as a desired outcome, but improved EOL care as evaluated by measuring outcomes that reflect quality end-of-life closure can help the public at large to see the dying process as a more positive part of life

    2.   Attention to realistic outcomes of care, better understanding and utilization of advanced directives, and increased use of hospice and palliative care services are strategies that can reduce costs at the end of life[1]

III. **The Role of the Nurse**

A. **Nurses as the constant across all settings**

    1.   Nurses are the health care providers who spend more time with the patients and their families than any other member of the health care team

    2.   Extending palliative care principles across settings to improve end of life care

    3.   Integrating palliative care principles across settings

        a)   Nurses enter into intense, intimate relationships with patients and families

        b)   They are therefore in a key position to impact patients' and families' ability to accomplish life completion goals by incorporating the principles of hospice and palliative care across all health care settings

4.   The American Nurses Association's *Code for Nurses*[21] emphasizes that "nursing care extends to anyone requiring the services of the nurse for the promotion of health, the prevention of illness, the restoration of health, the alleviation of suffering and the provision of supportive care of the dying"

5.   In any setting, the application of knowledge and skills that reflect the principles of palliative care allow the nurse to recognize subtle shifts in the patient's condition that often affect patient and family care preferences; this allows for timely reevaluation and resetting of goals

6.   Nurses can impact quality end-of-life closure by identifying persons with any life-threatening illness or condition

   a)   Early identification means that palliative care can be started sooner, allowing patients and families to set and achieve goals[4]

   b)   One very useful technique is to ask, "Is the patient now sick enough that it would not be a surprise if he/she died in the next 3–12 months?" This may identify patients who would otherwise not be recognized to be in need of palliative care[17]

B.   Expanding the concept of healing

1.   Ensuring quality EOL closure

   a)   At the end of life, nursing care shifts from a focus of wellness/recovery to an understanding of "healing"[22]

   b)   Because of their unique relationship to patients and families, nurses are in a position to promote comfort care for the dying as an active, desirable, and important skill, and an integral component of nursing care

2.   Healing

   a)   Comes from attention to the multiple dimensions that influence a person's quality of life[14]

   b)   Healing requires the recognition of the human face of each person and the communication that both the healer and the healed share a bond that ties them to each other through their humanity and their mortality[23]

C.   The Importance of "Presence"

1.   Some things cannot be "fixed"

   a)   Care at the end of life can frustrate health professionals, family and friends when attempts to decrease suffering are either not possible or interventions are not successful[9]

   b)   Some things that cannot be fixed[9, 24]:

      (1)   We cannot change the inevitability of death

      (2)   We cannot erase the anguish felt when someone we love dies

      (3)   We all must face the fact that we too will die

            (4)   No matter how hard we try, the perfect words or gestures to relieve patient and family distress rarely, if ever, exist

            (5)   It is often enough to just be with the person

    2.   The use of "Presence" as a way of expressing compassionate caring

        a)   To be present with dying patients and their families is to allow oneself to enter into another's world and to respond with compassion[25]

        b)   The nurse can use therapeutic presence as a means of communicating care for the patient struggling with the emotional and spiritual elements of suffering associated with multiple losses

        c)   "Presence may in fact be our greatest gift to these patients and their families"[26]

D.   Maintaining a realistic perspective

    1.   There is no right way to die, no cookbook approach

    2.   Crises and difficulties arise along with unexpected and profound joys

    3.   A flexible approach is essential to meet the changing needs of the patient and family

    4.   Recognition that quality of life (QOL) is determined by the unique needs of the patient and family assists the nurse in remaining focused on goals of care

IV.   The Nurse's Role in Improving Care Systems*

A.   Reasons to participate in and lead reform

    1.   Current services and reliability are woefully inadequate.

    2.   The best of current practices would not yield a competent, reliable care system for those "sick enough to die".

    3.   The special trust that society gives to health care professionals includes an obligation to ensure high quality, reliability, and pursuit of excellence

    4.   When the care system has especially serious shortcomings in serving its' community, professionals have similarly strong obligations to correct those shortcomings

    5.   Specific skills, attitudes, and behaviors are helpful in this work and they can (and should) be learned and taught

    6.   The history of reform in end of life care has been dominated by nursing—from establishing hospice programs through quality improvement projects; nurse leaders and managers have the opportunity and track record to make improvements happen

    7.   No one knows exactly how to put together trustworthy, reliable, effective and efficient care systems; the pace of useful change depends on the pace of learning, which largely depends on innovation, evaluation, and communication

---

* The source of this information is the ELNEC Curriculum, AACN & COH, (2000). Used with permission.

B. What would reform aim to do?

1. At the most general level, provide a care system that can promise to a person who has a life-limiting progressive illness:

   a) Good medical treatment

   b) Competent symptom management

   c) Continuity, coordination, and comprehensiveness

   d) Inclusion in the care-planning process

   e) Individualized care reflecting patient and family preferences

2. It helps to think of "the population of people who _____", rather than just the separate individual, i.e. not just how to help Mr. Smith, but also how to reliably and effectively serve patients like Mr. Smith

3. Nurses might conceive of improvement activities at various "levels": personal, service team, provider organization, region, state and federal policy

   a) Service Teams

   (1) The strongest vehicle for improvement seems to be rapid cycle quality improvement. Many variations are possible, but fundamental elements include[17]:

   (a) An aim—stated in demonstrable terms relevant to patients and "owned" by the team

   (b) A team that wants to achieve the aim and is willing to work to do so

   (c) A measure that will show whether the team is achieving the goal

   (d) A set of changes that might achieve the aim

   (e) Serial implementation of changes, with evaluation and learning, by the team, from each Plan-Do-Study-Act Cycle (PDSA cycle)

   (f) The expansion and implementation of effective changes, which sustains reform, and builds on success

   (2) One of the most difficult arenas for change is "noticing" or "attending to" deficits in care; nurses must become uncomfortable with routine shortcomings in order to develop motivation and commitment to change

   (3) Changes that might be seen as shortening a patient's life require careful attention; be sure that many people are involved and that good intentions and thoughtful considerations are well evidenced

   b) Provider organizations

   (1) Rapid cycle quality improvement (under various names) is central to improving organizational performance

   (a) The process is the same

   (b) Organizational leadership is often very important to sustained improvement

   (2) There is a strong track record of nurse-led success in improving end of life care when the team aims for improving performance in an arena that they "own"

    c)   Regional health care systems

        (1)   Most patients need the services of multiple organizations; promises need to be "durable" across time and organizations

        (2)   Very little work has addressed continuity of people, care plans, advance directives, or anything else across time and settings; yet, this is essential

            (a)   Nurses can encourage, contribute to, and collaborate with efforts to make transfers less frequent, less disruptive, and better supported

            (b)   Likewise, standardization of protocols and measures of success for populations are useful and worthwhile

        (3)   At the least, nurses should be familiar with the settings that their patients utilize at the end of life, including their personnel, practices and potentials (i.e. the nursing home nurse needs to sit-in on a hospice team, visit the hospital discharge nurse, etc.)

    d)   State and federal policies

        (1)   The United States society built a health care system around acute illness—aiming mainly for prevention and rescue. The demographics are now different. Most people face many months of living with slowly progressive disabling disease—which will eventually be fatal.

        (2)   Eventually, all reform runs into dysfunctional coverage, reimbursement, and regulation. Professionals have an obligation to act to correct these problems.

        (3)   Some resources for policy reform

            (a)   Americans for Better Care of the Dying, http://www.abcd-caring.org

            (b)   Partnership for Caring, http://www.partnershipforcaring.org

            (c)   National Hospice and Palliative Care Organization (NHPCO), http://www.nhpco.org

V.   Death and Dying in the Hospital Setting

A.   All staff trained to provide aggressive care to save life

    1.   CPR expected to be performed unless a specific order says otherwise

    2.   Goals are rigorous care, resuscitation and recovery

    3.   Hard to prepare the patient and family for death when intensive efforts are ongoing to save the life

    4.   Death in Acute-care settings seen as resulting from ineffective care

B.   Standard hospital policies and procedures typically inconsistent with palliative and hospice care approaches

    1.   Nurses are in the best position to help reform these policies because they are the core of the health care delivery system in the hospital

2. Whichever changes nursing addresses, they should include principles and domains of hospice and palliative care, specifically:

   a) Interdisciplinary approach

   b) Patient centered reports and rankings of quality of care

   c) Family support

   d) Functional status

   e) Continuity of care

   f) Spirituality

   g) Advance care planning

   h) Projected survival time and decisions regarding the aggressiveness of care

   i) Physical and emotional symptom management

   j) Grief and bereavement

   k) Communication among caregivers, patients, and families

C. **Facilitating a Good Death in the Hospital**

   1. Palliative Care Pathways and Standard Orders should be in place

   2. Symptom relief protocols and standing orders for the palliative care patient

   3. Palliative Care consultation teams should include

      a) Nursing leadership

      b) Interdisciplinary team members

      c) Referral mechanisms

      d) Case management to maintain continuity across all settings

      e) Around the clock accessibility

   4. Palliative Care Units

      a) Provide a familiar environment for patient and family

      b) All staff have training to care for the palliative care patient

      c) May have some drawbacks:

         (1) Members of the healthcare team on other units may not feel they "need" to learn palliative care principles

         (2) Continuity of care may be compromised when patients transferred between units

   5. Bereavement Programs and Services

      a) The death of the patient does not signal an end to the care provided which is typical in the acute-care setting

      b) Family are also included in the unit of care, these services can meet a currently unmet need in hospital-based deaths

c)   As an institution bereavement services can also include sending a sympathy note, providing bereavement resources, and the timing of mailing the hospital bill[27]

D.   Ongoing Education for Medical and Nursing Staff: Developing standardized protocols to help staff respond to commonly occurring events (e.g. advance care planning, pronouncement of death)

E.   The Intensive Care Unit presents its own challenges

1.   Shift in the focus of care can be as short as minutes, giving little time for nursing staff to prepare the patient and the family for death

2.   ICU physically not set up for many visitors for long periods of time

a)   This presents a challenge for the nurse but an issue that deserves close attention

b)   Patients should have the opportunity to be with their loved ones while they are dying if that is their wish

3.   Communication with family members

a)   Fast pace of the ICU makes this difficult and inconsistent

b)   Multidisciplinary teams to work with the family so that their needs are met

c)   Involve the family in providing care, to the extent possible

F.   Bereavement follow up programs

1.   Family contact by phone or mail monthly until the one-year anniversary of the death

2.   Also found to be useful for the health-care providers to cope with their loss[28]

VI.   The End of Life Patient in the Long Term Care Setting

A.   Epidemiology of Long Term Care residents

1.   Half of Americans who live to 65 years of age by 2030 will enter a nursing home before they die

2.   2/3 of persons who consider a nursing home their usual place of residence will remain in the nursing home until death

3.   According to the two most recent years of the National Mortality Follow-back Survey, the probability that a nursing home will be the site of death increased from 18.7% in 1986 to 20.0% by 1993

4.   Current health care trends are likely to promote the use of nursing homes as a site for terminal care

5.   Nursing home hospice population expanded from 7.7% of all Medicare hospice beneficiaries in 1989 to 17% in 1995

6.   Only 1% of the nursing home population enrolls in hospice care

7.   70% of nursing homes have no hospice patients[29]

B.   Hospice and Palliative care in Long Term Care Facilities

1.   A Long Term Care Facility is the home of the patient

2.   Staff members of a Long Term Care Facility are caregivers to patients

    a)   Showing and sharing respect and care

    b)   Giving appropriate and necessary information

    c)   Assisting in decision-making of patients/residents

    d)   Encouraging family members to participate in care of resident

3.   Long Term Care Facility Staff also are professional members of interdisciplinary team. A challenge for all to:

    a)   Balance needs of patient with family and staff

    b)   Recognize the needs of patient foremost rather than those of family or staff

C.   Goal of Hospice/Palliative Care in a Long Term Care Facility

1.   Provide optimal end-of-life care

2.   Identify residents who have been diagnosed with a life-limiting, progressive illness and meet their needs

3.   Potential patients might include (not an all inclusive listing)

    a)   Advanced Cancer patients

    b)   End-stage Diabetic patients

    c)   End-stage Pulmonary Disease patients

    d)   End-stage Cardiac/CHF patients

    e)   End-stage Alzheimer's patients

    f)   End-stage Renal patients

4.   For eligibility requirements for admission to Medicare Hospice benefits refer to Chapter X

5.   Delivering end-of-life care may be provided within the dual regulations of the Long Term Care facility and the hospice, if the care plan reflects hospice philosophy and is based on an assessment of the patient's needs and specific living arrangement in the Long Term Care Facility

    a)   Preauthorization of individualized plan of care by hospice is required for each long term care facility

    b)   The primary physician remains in charge and he works cooperatively with the interdisciplinary team

    c)   The primary physician generally continues medical care

    d)   The Hospice Medicare Benefit requires bereavement services to family

D. Agreements with Long Term Care Facilities

1. Formal, legal agreements

    a) Written contracts required by Medicare

    b) Contracts required may vary from state to state

    c) Negotiated by administrators

2. Informal agreements

    a) Administrative support needed

    b) Need excellent, ongoing communication among all members of team

    c) Maintaining up-to-date information for all on a Long Term Care Facility patient and his status to both parties[30]

    d) Ensure comfort care at the end of life

    e) Hospice/palliative care team augment nursing facility services available to the terminally ill patient

E. Educational Needs for Long Term Care Facility Staff

1. Needs Assessment

    a) Who needs to learn what

    b) What are the best learning tools for each particular individual/group?

        (1) Didactic

        (2) Role-playing/simulation

        (3) Interactive discussions

        (4) One to one teaching

        (5) Self-study

2. Suggested topics for teaching

    a) Hospice and Palliative Care concepts and philosophy

    b) Facilitation of an interdisciplinary team

    c) Collaboration with the Hospice/Palliative Care Team

        (1) Interdisciplinary Team

            (a) Members

            (b) Role of each

        (2) Blending of roles

        (3) Conflict resolution

d) Involvement of family as part of unit of care- becoming "Partners in Caring"

   (1) Building and maintaining relationships

   (2) Support of family (teach coping skills, etc.)

e) Decision-making process

f) Pain and symptom management and other physical care issues

g) Spiritual and/or religious needs of the dying patient

h) Ethical issues of the dying

i) Cultural and ethnic effects and impact on dying patient

j) Grief, loss, mourning and bereavement for the resident, family & staff

k) Psychosocial Issues of the Dying Resident

   (1) Loss of everything, especially independence and control

   (2) Transition from chronic status to terminally ill status

   (3) Feelings of relief/burden "ready to go"

   (4) End-of-Life decision making

   (5) Signs of denial, bargaining, anger, and acceptance

   (6) Signs of anxiety, depression, and fear

   (7) Family signs of guilt, remorse, anger, resentment

   (8) Family members who suddenly appear on the scene

   (9) Need and use of counseling for family when needed

   (10) Bereavement for family/caregiver

   (11) Communication issues among:

      (a) Healthcare providers

      (b) Patient

      (c) Families/caregivers

      (d) Types of Communication

         (i) Verbal

         (ii) Non-verbal

   (12) Need to be truthful with the terminally ill patient, at his level of understanding and need

F. **Documentation of hospice care in a Long Term Care Facility**

1. Must meet regulations for both agencies

2. Must indicate a coordination of the plan of care

3. Goals of Hospice and the Long Term Care Facility must agree

4. Hospice must manage the plan of care

G.   Clinical care of the dying patient in a Long Term Care Facility should model clinical care provided in a private residence

    1.   Comprehensive assessment of the patient

    2.   Continual evaluation

    3.   Appropriate pain and symptom management

    4.   Appropriate hydration/nutrition

    5.   Frequent and good oral care

    6.   Prevention of infection

    7.   Skin integrity

    8.   Bowel and bladder care

    9.   Preparation of patient and family for approaching death

    10.   Maintenance of dignity of each patient

H.   Collaborative approach of hospice/palliative care team and Long Term Care Facility staff

    1.   Shared expertise

    2.   Care for patient and family

    3.   Mutual support

    4.   Mutual learning

    5.   Shared resources for both organizations and patient/family

I.   Symptoms that may indicate resident needs for further screening for hospice/ palliative care

    1.   Decreasing appetite

    2.   Decreased mobility

    3.   Increased sleepiness and decreased alertness

    4.   Loss of interest in life

    5.   Expressed desire to die

    6.   Worsening symptoms of disease process or development of new symptoms

J.   Advantages of Partnership between Long Term Care Facility and Hospice/Palliative Care

    1.   For the resident/family

        a)   Access to end-of-life care in their place of residence

        b)   Access to those in need of end-of-life care

        c)   Access to Hospice Medicare Benefit

        d)   Medications for symptoms related to the terminal illness

        e)   Durable medical equipment

        f)   Aggressive pain and symptom management

g) Bereavement follow-up

h) Staff trained in end-of-life care

2. For the Long Term Care Facility

a) Mentoring resource

b) Training and education source

c) Decision making

d) Support of staff

e) Assistance with Advance directives

f) Reduction in utilization of acute care facility

g) Increase bond with the community

3. For the Hospice/Palliative Care team

a) Meet primary objective to increase quality of life provided for all persons receiving end-of-life care

b) Support primary caregiver's needs

c) Continued relationship with community

K. **Hospice Nurse Role in the Long Term Care Facility**

1. Develop a trusting, honest relationship with Long Term Care Facility staff and residents

2. Maintain good communication with the staff at all times

3. Be a teacher/mentor in a non-threatening manner

4. Be a resource person

5. Assist in maintaining care plans for both institutions so that they are in agreement with each other

6. Attend team meetings of both institutions

7. Maintain good communication with primary physicians

8. Note any new physician orders and add to the hospice orders

9. Keep Long Term Care Facility up-to-date on patient-related issues

10. Frequently reevaluate patient's condition to monitor disease progression

L. **Future Challenges for Hospice and Long Term Care Facilities**

1. Increase of co-morbid diseases leading to greater severity of illness within Long Term Care Facilities

2. Increase in number of terminally ill dementia patients in Long Term Care Facilities

3. Maintaining hospice services within the Long Term Care environment

4. Recognizing that more than one hospice may have patients in the same facility, therefore efforts should be taken to avoid confusion in delivery of care

5. Accessing appropriate level of care that is financially reasonable and avoids conflict of skill

6. Necessity of ongoing continuing education of Long Term Care staff about hospice philosophy and practices

7. Challenge of turnover of long term care staff; often preventing consistency of care to be maintained

8. Decisions needing to be made

   a) Establishing a specific hospice unit within facility

   b) Utilizing beds as available throughout the facility

9. Continual evaluation of end-of-life care provided in a Long Term Care Facility[31]

10. Challenge of conducting research in the Long Term Care environment

VII. Conclusion

A. Quality EOL care encompasses physical, psychological, social, and spiritual aspects and includes the patient and the family as the unit of care

1. These not only are defining features of the nursing role, but also support the philosophy and principles of hospice and palliative care as well as reflect the dimensions within the Quality of Life model

2. Because nurses cannot practice what they do not know; increased knowledge is essential to improved patient care

B. Palliative nursing is not only "doing for", but is also largely "being with" patients and families

C. Hospice and Palliative care is best provided by nurses functioning as part of an interdisciplinary team and is not defined by location, but rather by the care needs of the dying patient and family

REFERENCES

1. Field, M.J. and C.K. Cassel, *Approaching death: Improving care at the end of life*. 1997, Institute of Medicine Task Force: Washington, DC.

2. Saunders, C., *Forward, in Oxford textbook of palliative care,* D. Doyle, G. Hanks, and N. MacDonald, Editors. 1993, Oxford University Press: New York.

3. Corr, C.A., *Death in modern society,* in *Oxford textbook of palliative medicine,* D. Doyle, G.W.C. Hanks, and N. MacDonald, Editors. 1998, Oxford University Press: New York. p. 31–40.

4. Super, A., *The context of palliative care within progressive illness,* in *Textbook of palliative nursing,* B. Ferrell and N. Coyle, Editors. 2001, Oxford University Press: New York.

5. Rosenberg, H.M., S.J. Ventura, and J.D. Maurer, *Births and deaths United States, 1995*. 1996, Monthly Vital Statistics Report, Preliminary Data from the Centers for Disease Control and Prevention, National Center for Health Statistics.

6. Ventura, S.J., et al., *Births and deaths: Preliminary data for 1997*. 1998, National Center for Health Statistics: Hyattsville.

7. Administration on Aging, *Older population by age: 1900 to 2050*. 2000, Administration on Aging.

8. Emanuel, L., C. von Gunten, and F. Ferris. *The education for physicians on end of life care (EPEC) curriculum*. 1999. Washington, DC: American Medical Association.

9. Rando, T.A., *Grief, dying and death: Clinical interventions for caregivers*. 1984, Champaign, IL: Research Press.

10. Scanlon, C., D*efining standards for end-of-life care*. American Journal of Nursing, 1997. **97**(11): p. 58–60.

11. SUPPORT, S.P.I., *A controlled trial to improve care for seriously ill hospitalized patients: A study to understand prognoses and preferences for outcomes and risks of treatments (SUPPORT)*. Journal of the American Medical Association, 1995. **274**: p. 1591–1598.

12. National Hospice and Palliative Care Organization, *Press release: New findings address escalating end-of-life debate*. 1996, National Hospice and Palliative Care Organization: Alexandria.

13. Egan, K. and M.J. Labyak, *Hospice care: A model for quality end-of-life care,* in *Textbook of palliative nursing,* B.R. Ferrell and N. Coyle, Editors. 2001, Oxford University Press: New York. p. 7–26.

14. Byock, I.R., *Dying well: The prospects for growth at the end of life*. 1997, New York: Riverhead Books.

15. Ferrell, B., R. Virani, and M. Grant, *Analysis of end-of-life content in nursing textbooks*. Oncology Nursing Forum, 1999. **26**(5): p. 869–876.

16. National Hospice and Palliative Care Organization, *Hospice fact sheet*. 2000, National Hospice and Palliative Care Organization: Alexandria.

17. Lynn, J., J.L. Schuster, and A. Kabcenell, *Improving care for the end of life: A sourcebook for health care managers and clinicians*. 2000, New York: Oxford University Press.

18. Ferrell, B.R., G. Juarez, and T. Borneman, *Outcomes of pain education in community home care*. Journal of Hospice and Palliative Nursing, 1999. **1**(4): p. 141–150.

19. Teno, J., I.R. Byock, and M.J. Field, *Research agenda for developing measures to examine quality of care and quality of life of patients diagnosed with life limiting illness.* Journal of Pain and Symptom Management, 1999. **17**(2): p. 75–82.

20. Lagnado, L., *Rules are rules: Hospice's patients beat the odds, so Medicare decides to crack down,* in *The Wall Street Journal.* 2000: New York. p. A1, A18.

21. American Nurses Association, *Code for nurses with interpretive statements.* 1985, Kansas City, MO: American Nurses Association.

22. Coyle, N., *Introduction to palliative nursing,* in *Textbook of palliative nursing,* B.R. Ferrell and N. Coyle, Editors. 2001, Oxford University Press: New York. p. 3–6.

23. Sulmasy, D.P., *The healer's calling.* 1997, New York/Mahway: Paulist Press.

24. Yates, P. and K.M. Stetz, *Families' awareness of and response to dying.* Oncology Nursing Forum, 1999. **26**(1): p. 113–120.

25. O'Connor, P., *Clinical paradigm for exploring spiritual concerns,* in *Death and spirituality,* K.J. Doka and J. Morgan, Editors. 1993, Baywood Publishing Company: New York.

26. Borneman, T. and K. Brown-Saltzman, *Meaning in illness,* in *Textbook of palliative nursing,* B.R. Ferrell and N. Coyle, Editors. 2001, Oxford University Press: New York.

27. Whedon, M.B., *Hospital care,* in *Textbook of palliative nursing,* B. Ferrell and N. Coyle, Editors. 2001, Oxford University Press: New York.

28. Puntillo, K. and D. Stannard, *The intensive care unit,* in *Textbook of palliative nursing,* B. Ferrell and N. Coyle, Editors. 2001, Oxford University Press: New York.

29. Zerzan, J., S. Stearns, and L. Hanson, *Access to palliative care and hospice in nursing homes.* Journal of the American Medical Association, 2000. **284**(10): p. 2489–2493.

30. Jones, D.H., *Caring for hospice patients in a long term care facility.* Caring Magazine, 1993: p. 228–230.

31. Keay, T.J. and R.S. Schonwetter, *Hospice care in the long-term care facility.* American Family Physician, 1998. **56**: p. 491–494.

GENERAL REFERENCES

American Association of Colleges of Nurses. (1997). *A peaceful death.* (Report from the Robert Wood Johnson End-of-Life Care Roundtable). Washington, DC: Author.

Bookbinder, M. (2001). Improving the quality of care across all settings. In B.R. Ferrell, & N. Coyle (Eds.) *Textbook of palliative nursing.* New York: Oxford University Press.

Derby, S. & O'Mahony, S. (2001). Elderly patients. In B.R. Ferrell, & N. Coyle (Eds.) *Textbook of palliative nursing.* New York: Oxford University Press.

Flynn, J.F. (2000, June). Hospice services and long term care facilities. Unpublished presentation for Ohio area long term care facilities.

Health Care Financing Administration (HCFA). (2000). Medicare hospice benefits. Boston: Author.

Hinds, P.S., Oakes, L. & Furman, W. (2001). End-of-life decision making in pediatric oncology. In B.R. Ferrell, & N. Coyle (Eds.) *Textbook of palliative nursing.* New York: Oxford University Press.

Hughes, A. (2001). The poor and underserved. In B.R. Ferrell, & N. Coyle (Eds.) *Textbook of palliative nursing*. New York: Oxford University Press.

Kane, R.A. (1995). Ethical themes in long term care. In R.J. Katz, R.L. Kane & M.D. Mezey (Eds.). *Quality care in geriatric settings* (pp. 130–148). New York: Springer.

Kane, R.L. (1996). The evolution of the American nursing home. In R.H. Tinstock, L.E. Cluff, O. VonMering (Eds.). *The future of long term care: Social and policy issues* (pp. 145–168). Baltimore: Johns Hopkins University Press.

Oncolink. (1999, August 27). *Hospice in the long-term care facility.* University of Pennsylvania Cancer Center or access on-line at:
http://www.oncolink.upenn.edu/resources/hospitals/wissahickon/services/nursing.html

Rhymes, J.A. (1993). Hospice care in the long-term care facility. *Long Term Care Facility Medicine 1* (6): 14–24.

Smith, S.A. (2000). *Hospice concepts: A guide to palliative care in terminal illness.* Chicago: Research Press.

Sherman, D.W. (2001). Patients with acquired immune deficiency syndrome. In B.R. Ferrell, & N. Coyle (Eds.) *Textbook of palliative nursing*. New York: Oxford University Press.

Stanley, K.J. & Zoloth-Dorfman, L. (2001). Ethical considerations. In B.R. Ferrell, & N. Coyle (Eds.) *Textbook of palliative nursing*. New York: Oxford University Press.

Wilson, S.A. (2001). Long-term Care. In B.R. Ferrell, & N. Coyle (Eds.) *Textbook of palliative nursing*. New York: Oxford University Press.

Byock, I. (1996). The nature of suffering and the nature of opportunity at the end of life. *Clinics in geriatric medicine,* 12(2): 237–251.

Cassel, E. (1982). The nature of suffering and the goals of medicine. *New England Journal of Medicine,* 306(11): 639–645.

Curtis, J.R. & Rubenfeld, G.D. (2000). *Managing death in the ICU: The transition from cure to comfort.* Seattle, WA: University of Washington.

Doyle, D. Hanks, G.W.C., & MacDonald, N. (1998). Introduction. In D. Doyle, G. W.C. Hanks, & N. MacDonald (Eds.) *Oxford textbook of palliative care (2nd ed.)* (pp. 3–8). New York: Oxford University Press.

Ersek, M. (2001). The meaning of hope in the dying. In B.R. Ferrell, & N. Coyle (Eds.) *Textbook of palliative nursing*. New York: Oxford University Press.

Ferrell, B.R., & Coyle, N. (Eds.). (2001). *Textbook of palliative nursing*. New York: Oxford University Press

Ferrell, B. R. (1996). Humanizing the experience of pain and illness. In B. R. Ferrell (Ed.), *Suffering* (pp. 3–27). Sudbury, MA: Jones and Bartlett Publishers.

Frankl, V. E. (1984). *Man's search for meaning.* New York: Washington Square Press.

Highfield, M.E.F. (2000). Providing spiritual care to patients with cancer. *Clinical Journal of Oncology Nursing,* 4(3): 115–120.

Kahn, D. L., & Steeves, R. H. (1996). An understanding of suffering grounded in clinical practice and research. In B. R. Ferrell (Ed.), *Suffering*. Sudbury, MA: Jones and Bartlett Publishers.

Lair, G. S. (1996). *Counseling the terminally ill: Sharing the journey.* Washington, DC: Taylor & Francis.

Last Acts Task Force. (1997). *Precepts of palliative care.* Princeton, NJ: Robert Wood Johnson Foundation.

Matzo, M.L., & Sherman, D.W. (Eds.). (2001). *Palliative care nursing: Quality care to the end of life.* New York: Springer Publishing Company.

Speck, P. (1998). Spiritual issues in palliative care. In D. Doyle, G. W.C. Hanks, & N. MacDonald (Eds.) *Textbook of palliative care,* (pp. 805–814). New York: Oxford University Press.

Spross, J. A. (1996). Coaching and suffering. In B. R. Ferrell (Ed.), *Suffering* (pp. 3–27). Sudbury, MA: Jones and Bartlett Publishers.

Waller, A., & Caroline, N. L. (1996). *Handbook of palliative care in cancer.* Boston: Butterworth-Heinemann.

World Health Organization. (1990). Cancer pain relief and palliative care. *Technical Report Series 804.* Geneva, Switzerland.

Younger, J. B. (1995). The alienation of the sufferer. *Advances in Nursing Science,* 17(4): 53–72.

CHAPTER VIII

END-OF-LIFE CARE
FOR THE CHILD AND FAMILY

Lizabeth H. Sumner, RN, BSN

I. **Introduction**

    A. **This section is intended to provide hospice and palliative care nurses with a limited practical reference and some symptom management guidelines for adapting practice to the care of infants, children and adolescents with life-limiting, progressive illnesses**

    B. **It is assumed that the general practice of hospice or palliative nursing is adhered to based on the other sections in this curriculum**

    C. **Adaptations will be based on the age, developmental level, diagnosis and family specific circumstances**

    D. **Because the range of diagnoses for these infants and children is so varied, some important, generalized approaches will be offered that may cross many diagnoses**

II. **Common Pediatric Diagnoses seen in Hospice/Palliative Services**

    A. **Cancer[1]**

        1. These diagnoses continue to be the #2 cause of death overall for children 0–14 yrs of age

            a) Leukemia is most common form of childhood cancer

                (1) 80% are ALL, then AML is next highest in incidence of leukemia

                (2) History: Fever, bleeding, pain, and symptoms of anemia (fatigue/weakness/lassitude, pallor, dyspnea); symptoms of thrombocytopenia (petechiae, purpura, and bruising with minimal trauma); GI symptoms (anorexia, abdominal pain, and weight loss); symptoms of leukostasis/WBC clumping (headache, blurred vision, and respiratory problems due to leukemic infiltration of CNS and lungs); infections; generalized achiness

(3) Management: Follow CBCs, serum electrolytes (hyperkalemia, hypocalcemia, hyperuricemia, and hyperphosphatemia associated with grossly elevated WBC count and/or massive organ infiltration by leukemic cells); fever, bleeding patterns, infection patterns, neurological status changes, GI changes, Pulmonary changes, GU changes (painless gonadal swelling may indicate gonadal infiltrate), all pain and anxiety patterns

(4) Discuss with patient/family and physician the goals of treatments, desires regarding transfusing as a palliative goal for comfort or to prevent acute bleeds, increase energy

b)   Osteosarcoma—most common bone tumor in children

(1) History: original painful lesion in long bone (may or may not have been associated with soft tissue mass and/or local edema); history of lung metastases and respiratory dysfunction (commonest metastatic site); history related to other potential metastatic sites: bone, pleura, kidney, adrenal gland, brain, and pericardium; history of malaise, fatigue, fever, anorexia, weight loss, and pain

(2) Management: Follow systems noted above; follow changes in weight, changes in pain patterns, and fevers. Utilize a combined approach to pain for bone and tissue pain

c)   Rhabdomyosarcoma most common soft tissue cancer in children

(1) History: varies with anatomic location of tumor and the presence/extent of metastases; metastatic spread is via the blood and lymphatic systems, and frequent sites of spread are lung, bone, bone marrow, brain, spinal cord, lymph nodes, liver, heart, and breast; early spread within the muscle of origin and to adjacent tissue is common

(2) If orbital in origin: history of orbital invasion, ptosis, exophthalmos, cranial nerve involvement (especially nerves II, III, IV, and/or VI)

(3) If origin is non-orbital parameningeal sites: history of nasal obstructions, sinusitis, epistaxis, local pain, hypernasal speech, serous otitis media with facial palsy and conduction hearing loss; affected ear may have mucopurulent or sanguineous drainage; extension into meninges is common, with history of symptom of increased ICP. If ICP present child may have increased seizure activity and headaches

d)   Wilm's tumor: nephroblastoma-malignant embryonal neoplasm of kidney, typically effects younger children

(1) History: original abdominal mass and history of pain, fever, malaise, hematuria, possible hypertension due to cyclo activity; symptoms related to potential metastatic sites: lung, liver, brain, bone, and contralateral kidney

(2) Management: follow systems noted above; in addition, watch for symptoms related to compression of inferior vena cava; changes in fever and pain patterns

e)   Neuroblastoma

(1) History: original mass (usually abdominal, in adrenal gland or paraspinal ganglia; may occur in neck, paraspinal area of thorax, or pelvis); symptoms related to metastases; in order of occurrence, these are bone marrow, bone,

lymph nodes, liver, intracranial lesions from direct extension of bony sites in skull, skin, and testes; pain (especially bone pain, with high risk of pathologic fractures), abdominal masses—retroperitoneal lymph nodes; if thoracic masses, history of Superior Vena Cava (SVC) Syndrome, or Horner's Syndrome (miosis, ptosis, exophthalmos, anhidrosis); if any paraspinal involvement-spinal cord compression

    (2)   Management: follow systems noted above; also follow weight, watch for intractable diarrhea and/or hypertension (both rare); follow neuro status for acute cerebellar encephalopathy (also rare); monitor CBCs, serum electrolytes to influence decisions regarding treatment goals and observe for changes in pain patterns

  f)   Brain tumors

    (1)   Early signs/symptoms in child: irritability, lethargy, vomiting, anorexia, headache, papilledema, behavioral changes, bulging fontanels in infant

    (2)   Late signs/symptoms in child: increased intracranial pressure causing headache, vomiting, papilledema, increased irritability, decreased level of consciousness, changes in vital signs, including widening of pulse pressure, bradycardia, (slowed, irregular pulse), displacement of brain structures (herniation), seizures, personality changes, loss of sensation, disturbances in coordination, malnutrition and dehydration. Side effects of anticonvulsant therapy may lead to gum hypertrophy, bleeding, gingivitis and changes in self esteem due to change in appearance/Cushingoid syndrome.

    (3)   Unique issues: prognosis has not changed in last 10 years; many symptoms drastically affect normal functioning

2.   Spectrum of cancer in children differs markedly from that in adults

  a)   Childhood cancer: usually involves hematopoetic system, nervous system and connective tissue

  b)   Neuroblastoma, Wilm's tumor, retinoblastoma, hepatoma rarely occur in adults[2]

B. Non-cancer diagnoses[1]

1.   Congenital anomalies

  a)   Account for the third highest cause of death in children 0–14 and create the largest group of children who could benefit from a hospice or palliative care program and include:

    (1)   Trisomy 13 and 18

    (2)   Osteogenesis Imperfecta Type II

    (3)   Werdnig Hoffman, Walker-Warburg Syndrome

    (4)   Anencephaly

    (5)   Holoprosencephaly

    (6)   Severe hydrocephaly

    (7)   Cardiac anomalies not compatible with life or determined to be inoperable/ surgery not elected

        b)   Pathophysiology

            (1)   Two Major Types

                (a)   Malformations, arising during embryogenesis (e.g. anencephaly)

                (b)   Deformations, late changes in previously normal structures due to pathologic processes or intrauterine forces (e.g. hydrocephalus)

            (2)   1/3 are "inherited" anomalies (spontaneous gene or chromosomal mutations)

            (3)   1/3 are multifactoral (including toxic/environmental factors)

            (4)   1/3 are of unknown causes

    2.   Muscular diseases include Muscular Dystrophy or Spinal Muscular Atrophy; Metabolic disorders; late stage Cerebral Palsy has significant muscular involvement

    3.   Children who have been profoundly injured or had a sudden acute illness event and will not have life support continued for prolonged period should be identified for hospice consultation and support

    4.   Other relevant conditions include metabolic/mitochondrial disorders, Tay Sachs, Intrauterine or birth related trauma/events, i.e. Hypoxic Ischemic Encephalopathy (HIE)

C.   Perinatal hospice

    1.   A prenatal diagnosis of a potentially lethal condition can be the catalyst for a hospice referral to support the expectant parents and other family throughout the pregnancy, labor and delivery

    2.   "Traditional" hospice support and care for the baby if he/she survives the immediate time of delivery

    3.   Grief support in anticipation of the possibility of death and Bereavement support for the family when the baby dies and afterwards

    4.   Includes the same preventative approach to minimize physical, emotional and spiritual suffering and to prevent the initiation of unintended, undesired, or futile interventions; emphasis is on *Quality of life* and creating opportunities for a personalized, family centered experience, regardless of the duration of the baby's life

III. Differences between Pediatric and Adult Hospice Care

A.   Pediatric Issues[3]

    1.   Not legally able to make decisions regarding treatment; yet want to participate in decisions; assent versus consent

    2.   The child's needs may be perceived differently by parents than by the sick child or staff thus affecting provision of care and communication

    3.   May not have verbal skills to adequately express feelings and needs

    4.   Have varied conceptions of and reactions to illness and death based on the following factors: age, developmental level; family/religious/cultural norms; cognitive, intellectual and emotional maturity

5.   Has not achieved a "full and complete life"

6.   Desire a sense of "normalcy" and typically prefer to be at home versus hospital

B.   Family Issues[3]

1.   Financial stressors: one or both parents may need to keep working, resulting in an inadequate support system

2.   Respite often needed from being around-the-clock caregivers

3.   Parents and staff must deal with sibling's feelings, which may include: acting out, anger, regressive behavior, anticipatory grief, fear, and/or problems at school

4.   Fear of being alone and/or feelings of helplessness with responsibility of caring for their dying child

5.   Adults often feel the need to protect the sick child and/or siblings by withholding information regarding diagnosis, treatment and/or prognosis

6.   Parental belief that "there must be something more that can be done"

C.   Community/Agency Issues[3]

1.   Must provide ongoing staff support and education regarding staff's own grief and personal issues

2.   Lack of referrals from physicians hesitant to stop "curative" treatment, who may believe they have "failed the child and family"

3.   Reimbursement for pediatric hospice care may be difficult to obtain and can be more costly than adult care

4.   Assessment of "Hospice appropriateness" of 6 months or less may be difficult to determine

5.   Need ongoing commitment of agency to pediatric program in spite of small pediatric hospice population

D.   Staff Issues[3]

1.   Must be knowledgeable regarding physical assessment, pain and symptom management for infants and children, and pediatric disease processes

2.   Staff may project fears for own children onto pediatric patient and family, i.e., "If it were my child..." They should..."

3.   Must be able to recognize developmental level of child regarding cognitive understanding about death and dying

4.   Need education on the real needs of dying children i.e. children feel pain, want honest information and worry about their condition and its effects on others; be able to focus on "the living" yet to be done within the context of the child's limitations

IV. General Issues Related to Admission of Pediatric Patients

A. Family centered approach to care.

1. Requires an interdisciplinary, collaborative team approach that focuses first and foremost on the needs of the *whole* FAMILY as a unit, to enable them to optimally thrive and cope within the context of the child's condition as it changes over time

2. Creates an inclusive model that optimally benefits the family and child, as the team works together to meet *their* goals for care and for *living*

3. Typically requires a broader scope of individuals and providers, beyond the "patient/caregiver" model for adult hospice care

    a) *Whole* family care involves support and intervention for all of the family as the needs arise. May include the child's school as indicated or that of the sibling(s)

    b) May include Child Life Specialist, multiple medical specialists and ancillary staff such as PT, OT, play therapy, music or art therapy etc.

4. Sets a standard of involving the siblings in ongoing discussions and supports helping them understand the child's condition and clarify their perceptions of cause and expression of fears and concerns

    a) Siblings need to be included in the circle of care and their individual emotional, developmental and basic needs met throughout the illness and into bereavement

    b) Feeling validated and supported during the sibling's illness and offering ways for the child to participate in the experience may assist him/her in adaptation during the illness and after child's death

B. Identify existing supports

1. Determine what is available and also what is needed for the ill child's and/or sibling's school community as the child enrolls in hospice/palliative care and as condition progresses, through child's death

2. Collaborate with the social worker to maintain contact with child's school, mechanism for classmate contact (counselor, teacher etc.)

3. Identify all who are directly contributing to the child's plan of care; may be multiple sites or providers

C. Identify the existing spiritual and or religious influences and supports for the child, siblings and parents belief system

D. Treatment/intervention goals

1. Discuss with child's primary MD and parents (and child as developmentally appropriate/physically capable)

    a) Goals for treatment therapies

    b) Goals that each person has, including the child to the extent possible

    c) Use each change in condition or new symptom as an opportunity to review child/family goals.

2.   This discussion is essential to articulate as much as possible, the intent, benefit, burden, and *meaning* of the treatments for all involved

3.   Upon discussion it may become evident that the understanding and perceptions of the goals of treatments may be shared, divergent or conflicting among those involved

   a)   Some interventions may be considered for continuation

   b)   Others may be "titrated" down in intensity

   c)   Other interventions may not be consistent with mutually agreed upon goals or are no longer contributing to quality of life for the child

4.   When creating a plan of care with the child/family, it is very important to place emphasis on the parent's *desired intensity of care* and symptom management for the child

   a)   This requires a thoughtful, planned discussion with consideration of timing and the readiness of parents

   b)   Key caregivers must participate

   c)   Provide an appropriate setting for the discussion

   d)   Be sure that adequate information is available

E.   Pain and symptom management: this section specifically highlights those distinctly different issues related to children and suggestions for helpful approaches

1.   Thoroughly assess medical, psychosocial, spiritual needs and issues of the sick child, parents, siblings, and even grandparents when involved directly

2.   QUESTT[4]:

   a)   **Q** = Question the child. Verbal statement/description of pain is most important factor in pain assessment

   b)   **U** = Use pain rating scales. Provides subjective quantitative measure of pain intensity

   c)   **E** = Evaluate behavior. Common indicators of pain in children and are especially valuable in assessing pain in non-verbal children, including infants

   d)   **S** = Secure parent's involvement because they know their child best

   e)   **T** = Take cause of pain into account because pathology or procedure may give clues to expected intensity and type of pain

   f)   **T** = Take action to meet the established goal (child's acceptable pain level) because the only reason to assess pain is to be able to relieve it through use of analgesic/adjuvant drugs and/or non-pharmacological methods

3.   GOLDEN RULE: Whatever is painful to an adult is painful to a child or an infant!

4.   Utilize EMLA cream for blood draws or IV insertion to decrease distress or fears.

5.   Detailed guides for pain and symptom management in hospice and palliative care are found in Chapters IV and V

6.   Safe and effective pain management is essential regardless of age and size of infant or child.

F.   After-hours coverage and continuity of care

1.   Needs of child/family should to be assessed prior to admission to either hospice or palliative care program

a)   Consider if and how the individual hospice/palliative care program can meet anticipated needs

b)   If needs cannot safely and realistically be met with the present resources, identify additional or alternative resources in the community best equipped to handle and meet the pediatric patient/family needs

c)   Attempt to create a collaborative framework to meet the needs of patient and family with all providers involved with child's care/family needs.

2.   For children and their families, a high priority must be placed on Continuity of care

a)   Fragmented or poorly coordinated care for the child and family can exacerbate an already strained coping pattern

(1)   The nurse can facilitate communication between the providers and the family in order to maintain the established plan of care for the child/family and to avoid frustration, confusion and duplication of efforts

(2)   Maximizing opportunities to communicate between providers and ensure continuity between settings (home, clinic, hospital, school etc) is an important and primary role of the nurse

b)   As a "case manager" the nurse can keep the team and other healthcare providers updated on the evolving plan of care for the child and keep the existing support system intact for the benefit of the family

c)   Regular reports to referral sources can maintain optimal contact with the child's care team

V.   Developmental Considerations in Pediatric Assessment

A.   Special considerations for examining and interpreting assessment information are necessary for clinicians dealing with infants and children[5]

B.   Appraisal of the child's developmental level is the first step toward a positive interaction, which reinforces the child's sense of security, mastery and self-esteem

1.   **Infant (0–1 year)**

a)   Stranger anxiety is prevalent at 7 months of age and older; do physical examination with parent holding baby or within close view; smile; approach should be unhurried and gentle, use high pitched, soft voice; avoid abrupt jerky movements

b)   Pain related behaviors: increased irritability, changes in crying patterns, handling/feeding changes, usual comfort measures less effective, facial expression is vigilant or angry, withdraws affected body part

(1)   In the first few months there is no apparent "understanding" of pain but baby has response to painful stimuli

(2)   Children eventually develop anticipatory fear related to perceived painful situations, and as verbal skills develop uses descriptive words for pain such as "owie, boo-boo, ouchie"

(3)   Ask parent/child how pain/hurt is referred to; utilize the familiar words for pain in the family; plan supportive interventions with parents; child may withdraw from social or play activity if pain persists.[5]

2.   **Toddler (1–3 years)**

a)   Separation and stranger anxiety decreases by age two

b)   Examine child in parent's lap, complete physical assessment through playful interactions (i.e. "Simon Says..." and puppet play) and minimize initial physical contact

c)   Praise for cooperative behavior

d)   Identify words used for pain and discomfort

e))   Offer choices when appropriate

3.   **Preschool Child (3–5 years)**

a)   Likes being a "helper", having choices and trying out equipment for him/herself; fearful of bodily harm

b)   Examine with parent close by

c)   Needs positive reinforcement and praise

d)   Less tentative than toddlers

e)   Identify words used by child to describe pain

f)   Offer choices when appropriate and incorporate measures that the child believes will work such as warm wash cloth on abdomen[5]

4.   **School-age Child (5 years+)**

a)   Able to understand simple explanations regarding illness and body functioning

b)   Developing understanding of "cause and effect", understands relationship between pain, other symptoms and disease process

c)   Provide age appropriate information and teaching regarding pain regimen and rationale

d)   Answer questions briefly and honestly

e)   Include child in decision making process when possible

f)   Identify words to describe pain used by child

g)   Utilize dolls for "parallel" assessment and intervention

h)   Use appropriate picture books for aiding in explanation of bodily functions or changes.

i)   Offer choices when appropriate and incorporate measures that the child believes will work

5. **Adolescent**

    a) More privacy and independence needed, prefers being included in explanation/findings

    b) More introspective; increasing use of mental/cognitive coping strategies; has capacity for coherent understanding of physiologic processes

    c) Allow for adolescent's input, insight and choices

    d) Attention needs to given to self esteem and personal image as it changes over time, related to peers and develop strategies to assuage distress in this area, reinforce the positives and choices available

    e) Participation in decision-making may be influenced by culture, age and religious norms of family

VI. General Care Issues for Child/Family

A. Symptom management approaches

1. Nurse needs to be familiar with the child's developmental level to engage in any discussion on how they are physically feeling, for teaching related to care or disease progression, selection of pain assessment tools

2. Give child and parents choices in planning medication, treatments or procedures and their daily living regimen to fit family lifestyle and goals for comfort

3. An important element of care for children and their families is the maintenance of NORMALCY in as many areas of life as possible and the incorporation of attention to physical appearance/self-esteem into daily routines

4. CONTROL is a most important aspect of approaching care for both the child and parents

    a) The sick child may demonstrate an increased need for structure and routine as their scope of control diminishes

    b) This is normal and should be accommodated with an ongoing attempt to give choices and respect their need for routine that reinforces a sense of safety and security

5. Nursing visits typically involve some socialization activities with the child and siblings to create a therapeutic and relaxed environment prior to doing physical exam as a means of transitioning focus of time together

    a) Child will be more at ease when related to as a child first and as a sick child last

    b) Incorporate play into methods of communication

    c) Assume a relaxed posture, perhaps sitting beside the child on the floor, at his/her level, having "child friendly" clothes and demeanor

B. Planning care for the Pediatric patient

1. This patient population requires familiarity with and a planned response to any potential symptoms for the child's disease process and diagnosis (See Appendix 3: Standards of Hospice Care for Children)

2. Identify those symptoms or perceived "emergencies" which the child and parents fear most and have a plan in place to respond quickly to treat them across possible settings (home, hospital, school, Palliative Care unit, inpatient hospice)

3. Nurses need to anticipate and prepare a plan for these to prevent and minimize experience of suffering fear or pain

4. Examples may include:

    a) Seizure management: have necessary medications in appropriate routes on hand for children with any neurological component to their disease to respond to any possible seizure symptoms, which may cause physical or emotional distress (suggestions include: Lorazepam, Gabapentin, Phenobarbital, Phenytoin, Diazepam, Diastat)

    b) Pain management is essential for **all** ages

        (1) Select appropriate routes and dosages *based on weight (mg/kg)* for infants and children

        (2) Discuss with and provide education to parents and child on safe use, benefits of narcotics/opioids for pain relief and what to expect

            (a) Assist them to create a schedule that fits their lifestyle and maintains desired level of relief

            (b) Consider cultural and ethnic influences as well as the exposure to education in schools related to illegal drug use (DARE programs etc), which may influence perception of the use of therapeutic medications

        (3) Consider combined strategies and/or methods for complex pain and multiple types of pain

        (4) Assess for pain in the non-verbal child with behavioral indicators and facial expressions, appropriate pain assessment tools. Examples include:[4]

            (a) Poker chip tool (how many pieces of pain do you have?)

            (b) Eland color tool (selection of colors to represent intensity of pain applied to outline image of child's body)

            (c) Faces scale (series of 5 faces to represent range of pain ratings); Numeric scales (usually 1–5 or 1–10)

        (5) Pain in children can be approached with the principles of the WHO ladder as it applies to all patients

    c) Anxiety and agitation

        (1) Minimizing stress and anxiety in the child relieves the suffering and anxiety of parents as well

        (2) Agitation may arise related to tests and procedures, strangers, previous experiences, untreated/undertreated pain, and from fears related to his/her condition, one's future, concerns for self or family, what will happen as they are dying, etc.

        (3) Pharmacologic and non-pharmacologic interventions should be used such as relaxation/soothing strategies; Lorazepam, diazepam, reassess pain regimen for efficacy

d) Respiratory difficulties, dyspnea, congestion

  (1) These can be very distressful to caregivers/parents and cause restlessness in the child

  (2) Using medication to decrease secretions may benefit the child (glycopyrrolate [Robinul®], scopolamine patch)

  (3) Assess fluid intake versus volume tolerated

    (a) May need to adjust feedings if congestion continues

    (b) Parents may need education on the symptoms of fluid overload, the inability to tolerate routine feedings in the child's current condition

    (c) Gradually decreasing fluids based on demand and tolerance is easier for parents than an all or none approach

    (d) Trial use of oxygen may be beneficial if it does not increase agitation (use pediatric cannula or mask or blow by)

e) Elimination

  (1) Maintain bowel function and prevent the acute stress and distress associated with constipation and the need for invasive remedies

  (2) Invasive efforts to relieve constipation are very traumatic and risky for the child especially the oncology patient with bleeding precautions

  (3) PREVENTION is very important via nutrition, hydration and a preventative bowel regimen to avoid painful stooling/constipation. Hydration as long as possible to maintain urination, avoid indwelling catheters and maintain general comfort and hygiene

f) Blood products/transfusions

  (1) Pediatric patients often benefit from continuing intermittent transfusions if they add to or maintain a desired quality of life; may help the child to accomplish specific personal goals, i.e. graduation, birthday, significant outing or other milestone etc.

  (2) These interventions may prevent a traumatic dying experience if it is expected that the child may actually hemorrhage or will die at home with that possibility

  (3) The balance of benefit/burden for these therapies and the decision whether or not to provide them is a discussion to plan ahead for and review over time as the child's condition changes to review the goals for care

g) Depression

  (1) May not be anticipated in the dying child or adolescent, but needs to be assessed when symptoms appear

  (2) Children show the same symptoms as adults, i.e., becoming more withdrawn, apathy for known interests, decreased tolerance to change and increased labile emotions, irritability, sleep disorders, etc.

  (3) Consult with physician, social worker, psychologist or psychiatrist to determine the best pharmacologic approach

(4) Reassure parents and child that depression is treatable and not uncommon

(5) Utilize immediate onset medications for a more rapid therapeutic effect

C. Preparation for the last days of life

1. Utilize hopeful language in context of condition

   a) Negative and consistently "death oriented" discussions are not palatable for most children and their families on a regular basis

      (1) Parents are often not prepared to make final arrangements until death is imminent or afterwards

      (2) This may not be denial, but rather a personal decision reflecting the parents' needs and beliefs

   b) "Titrate" family's ability to handle these discussions, as trust and readiness are apparent

      (1) Forcing them may lead to conflict and hostility or even rejection of care

      (2) Hope is always present in some form and some expression for these families

2. As much as possible, plan where the death will take place

   a) With the help and support of the Interdisciplinary team, discuss with patient and parents where they would prefer the death to occur

   b) Explore any fears or concerns—realistic or not—related to the decisions for place of death and dispel if appropriate

   c) Communicate the plan to all staff involved, especially those that cover after hours, at change of shift or assignments etc.

3. Explore and discuss the spiritual dimension of the child's life as it relates to coping with their illness and life changes

   a) Have similar discussions with each parent and the sibling(s) and grandparents, if present

   b) Collaborate with chaplain/spiritual counselor to address the needs and concerns that arise during these discussions

      (1) Discuss what would bring comfort at this time and what continues to be a source of strength to each of them.

      (2) Facilitate obtaining the desired spiritual and or religious support

      (3) Provide for rituals requested

4. Prepare family members and child as he/she desires for what to expect as the dying process nears

   a) Providing this in a written form is particularly helpful for them to refer to and to use with other relatives

   b) Use language that is gentle, informative and based on child's level of understanding

VII. Counsel/Provide Emotional Support for Child's Grief

A. **Important to consider developmental stages as the context upon which to base explanations, education, needs assessment and relevant approaches.**

1. If children have a sibling or a parent, significant grandparent etc who is dying, the issues of their grief need to be assessed and addressed by the IDT

2. IDT members, including the nurse have significant opportunities to make the child feel included, to validate concerns and anticipatory grief, their desire to help and participate fulfilled—PRIOR to the death of their loved one

3. Grieving begins upon the realization something is seriously wrong/has changed in the family and that "someone is not getting better."

B. **Eric Erikson's stages of human development; all stages are considered a "crisis" that must be overcome and mastered; non-resolution of a stage may handicap a person in later life; most marked effect on later life is the non-resolution of stage one: trust versus mistrust[6]**

1. Eric Erikson's stages

   a) Trust versus mistrust (infancy)

   b) Autonomy versus shame and doubt (early childhood)

   c) Initiative versus guilt (preschool)

   d) Industry versus inferiority (childhood)

   e) Identity versus diffusion (adolescence); directed toward dating and social roles

   f) Intimacy versus isolation (young adulthood)

   g) Generativity versus self-absorption (adulthood); most potential to change society

   h) Integrity versus despair (maturity)

2. Piagetian stages[7, 8]

   a) Sensory-motor (birth to 3 years): Infant goes through several substages that lead from complete self involvement to learning through trial and error to use certain acts to affect an object or a person; by age 2, toddler learns that certain actions have a specific effect on the environment; thinking is egocentric (for instance, if mother leaves, child thinks it is because of his/her action)

   b) Pre-operational (3–7 years): Thought is intuitive and prelogical (magical); thinking remains egocentric with conclusions based on what child feels or would like to believe

   c) Concrete operational thought (7–12 years): Conceptual organization becomes more stable and rational; child develops a conceptual framework that is used to evaluate and understand objects in the world around him/her

   d) Formal operational thought (12–18 years): Adolescent is increasingly able to deal effectively with reality, abstract thinking and future thinking; deductive reasoning develops; important ideals and attitudes develop in late adolescence

C. **Children and grief responses by age (note: children and adolescents do not grieve in a linear pattern but rather in a "clumping pattern" of sometimes intense periods separated by long intervals where they apparently are not affected by the loss)**[9]

1. The infant: birth to 2 years (pre-verbal)

   a) Grief reactions: irritability, change in crying or eating patterns, bowel or bladder disturbances, emotional withdrawal and slowing of development; clinginess; do not tolerate changes in daily living routines

   b) How to help: provide secure and stable environment, lots of TLC; follow a schedule, hold and play with the child often; a consistent caregiver and maintaining routines is critical

2. The preschool child: age 3 to 5 years

   a) Grief reactions: grasp of SOME concepts related to death, time and permanence are limited and often see death as temporary; may see seemingly inappropriate questions ("why can't we just go out and get another mom?"), indifference, physiological symptoms (sleeping, eating, stomach aches), regression, fears, imagined guilt/feelings of responsibility, wide-ranging emotions

   b) How to help: same as above; understand and accept the behavior as normal; use the correct terminology; BRIEF EXPLANATIONS; reassure the child he/she had nothing to do with CAUSING the ILLNESS OR the death

3. The grade school child: age 6 to 10

   a) Grief reactions: a child of this age gradually begins to understand death, but may still believe that it only happens to other people; may feel guilt (magical thinking) and blame self for death; may see on again, off again grieving, problems in school (including socially inappropriate behavior, anger towards teacher or classmates, poor grades, physical ailments), anger; at this age children are at the most risk for complicated grief—they intellectually understand death, but lack coping skills to deal with the emotions

   b) How to help: same as above; provide simple, honest, and accurate information, accept behavior as normal, contact and ask for help from school counselors and teachers, acknowledge normalcy of anger and teach ways to constructively express it

4. The pre-adolescent and adolescent: age 10 to 18

   a) Grief reactions: typically, by age 12 to 14, children have a complete view of mortality; they may, however, deny that death can happen to them or one of their peers; may view death as punishment; grief at this developmental stage may interfere with the child's development of identity; may see hidden or denied emotions, so called "common and normal adolescent behaviors" may be made worse by a loss at this stage (fighting, unruliness at school, rebellion, using drugs, sexual activity, suicidal tendencies)

   b) How to help: same as above; acknowledge that adolescents are not adults, and do not need to act or think like adults; evaluate supports available and informed at school; engage school and other trusted adults for support, be aware of destructive behaviors and set limits. Continue discipline parameters to maintain appropriate behavioral limits-this actually enhances security in the adolescent. Due to the inherent ambivalence and duality of feelings, intense emotions and desires for independence and tentativeness to release feelings; peer influences; may be interested in journaling, peer groups, tape recording, artistic expression, art therapy modes of expression

5.   Young adult: age 19 and over

    a)   Grief reactions: fully formed notion of death including how death affects him/her and changes in the family structure; may experience ambivalence and confusion about what is next for them, including the feeling of responsibility to take on some of the roles of the dead family member

    b)   How to help: urge the young adult to focus on their needs and be able to express them to adults around them as well as peers so that others can support them; may be interested in support groups (not easy in the midst of the pain of grief!)

D.   **Ten Needs of Grieving Children[10] ***

1.   **Adequate Information**

    a)   Children need information that is clear and comprehensible

    b)   When they don't have sufficient information, they'll make up a story to fill in the gaps

    c)   If possible children should be informed about an impending death; they already know something is taking place

    d)   They can become anxious, maybe feel responsible or may even wonder if they can "catch" whatever the cause of the person's death

2.   **Fears and Anxieties Addressed**

    a)   Children need to know they will be cared for; many children who lose one parent fear the other will die too; they fear for their own safety as well

    b)   Research has also shown that bereaved children who were given consistent discipline after parental death were less anxious than those for whom discipline became lax

3.   **Reassurance They Are Not to Blame**

    a)   Bereaved children may wonder, "Did I cause it to happen?" They need to know they didn't cause the death out of their anger or shortcomings

    b)   Younger children especially may experience "magical thinking" and may have difficulty in this area

4.   **Careful Listening**

    a)   Children need to have a person who will hear out their fears, fantasies, and questions and not minimize their concerns

    b)   Some of their questions may be uncomfortable for adults, yet they need answered as valid things kids wonder about

---

* Adapted by San Diego Hospice

5. **Validation of Individual's Feelings**

   a)   It is sometimes a temptation to tell a child how he or she should feel, but children's feelings must be acknowledged and respected as valid

   b)   Children also need to express their thoughts and feelings in their own way

   c)   Adults must remember each child's personality is unique as well as their relationship with the deceased

6. **Help with Overwhelming Feelings**

   a)   Children need help in dealing with emotions that are too intense to be expressed

   b)   The most common feelings expressed by bereaved children are sadness, anger, anxiety, and guilt

   c)   Sometimes these feelings are acted out, and adults can help kids express them in safer ways through play activities and/or writing

7. **Involvement and Inclusion**

   a)   Children need to feel important and involved before the death as well as afterward

   b)   It is recommended that children over age 5 be allowed to make an informed decision as to whether or not they want to attend the funeral, for example

   c)   Children may want to have something special they have made buried with the person

   d)   Children also need to be included in rituals around anniversaries or other special times when it's appropriate to remember the deceased in a more formal way

8. **Continued Routine Activities**

   a)   Children need to maintain age appropriate interest and activities

   b)   Adults sometimes need to be reminded that children cope and communicate through play activity (kids are kids first and grievers second)

9. **Modeled Grief Behaviors**

   a)   Learning theory tells us that modeled behavior is one of the most effective sources of learning; children learn how to mourn by observing mourning behavior in adults

   b)   Encouraging children to think about, to remember, and to talk about the deceased is a rather simple but effective way that adults can influence the course of bereavement in children

   c)   Acknowledging and sharing feelings with the child in this way is very important

10. **Opportunities to Remember**

   a)   Children need to be able to remember and to memorialize their lost loved one not only after the death but also continuously as they go through the remaining stages of life

   b)   Pictures and objects belonging to the deceased can be useful reminders of who the person was and the things that were important in the relationship; shared reminiscences can also be helpful

REFERENCES

1. Berry, P., K. Zeri, and K. Egan, *The hospice nurses study guide: A preparation for the CRNH candidate.* 2nd Edition ed. 1997, Pittsburgh, PA: Hospice Nurses Association.

2. American Cancer Society, *Cancer facts and figures 2000.* 2000, American Center Society.

3. Children's Hospice International, *Children's Hospice International: 2001 informational overview.* 2001, Children's Hospice International: Alexandria.

4. Wong, D.L., *Wong & Whaley's clinical manual of pediatric nursing.* 5th ed. 2000, St. Louis: Mosby.

5. Clark, E., *Palliative pain and symptom management for children and adolescents.* 1985, Children's Hospice International and Division of Maternal and Child Health—US Department of Health and Human Services: Alexandria.

6. Erikson, E., *Childhood and society.* 1963, New York: W.W. Norton & Co.

7. Wadsworth, B., *Piaget's theory of cognitive development.* 1971, New York: David McKay Co.

8. Petrillo, M. and S. Sanger, *Emotional care of hospitalized children: An environmental approach.* 2nd ed. 1980, Philadelphia: J.B. Lippincott.

9. Volker, B., *Hospice and Palliative Nurses Practice Review.* 3rd Edition ed, ed. B. Volker. 1999, Dubuque, IA: Kendall/Hunt Publishing.

10. Worden, J.W., *Children and grief: When a parent dies.* 1996, New York: The Guilford Press.

GENERAL REFERENCES

Armstrong-Daily, A. & Goltzer, S. (Eds.). (1993). *Hospice care for children.* New York: Oxford University Press.

Foley, G., Fochtman, D., & Mooney, K. (Eds.). (1993.) *Nursing care of the child with cancer.* (2nd ed.). Philadelphia: W.B. Saunders.

Hess, C.S. (1996). *The child in pain.* In D.L. Wong, W*ong and Whaley's Clinical Manual of Pediatric Nursing,* 4th Ed. St. Louis, MO: Mosby. pp. 314–331

RECOMMENDED RESOURCES

Borne, M.A. (1996). *The Harriet Lane Handbook.* (4th Ed.). Johns Hopkins Hospital. St. Louis, MO: C.V. Mosby.

ChIPPS. (2000). *Compendium of pediatric palliative care: Professional development and resource series.* Alexandria, VA: NHPCO.

Doka, K. (Ed.). (1995). *Children mourning/mourning children.* Washington, DC: Hospice Foundation of America.

Doyle, D., Hanks, G.W.C., & MacDonald, N. (Eds.). (1998). *Oxford textbook of palliative medicine.* (2nd Ed.). New York: Oxford University Press.

Ferrell, B.R. & Coyle, N. (Eds.). (2001). *Textbook of palliative nursing.* New York: Oxford University Press.

Texas Cancer Council. (2000). *End of life care for children.* Austin, TX: Author.

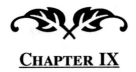

CHAPTER IX

INDICATORS OF IMMINENT DEATH

Kathy Kalina, RN, BSN
Joanne E. Sheldon, RN, MEd, CHPN, CIC

I. **Introduction**

A. **The last days and hours of life pose many challenges and opportunities for all involved with the dying person**

1. According to the literature, a majority of people do not have a death characterized by symptoms that are well controlled[1]

2. The signs and symptoms of an imminent death and their frequency vary with each patient and each diagnosis

3. Teach the family and/or caregivers that the patient may experience any number of the symptoms discussed below, or none

B. **Hospice and Palliative Care nurses must be experts at identifying the physical, spiritual and emotional signs and symptoms of imminent death. It is the responsibility of the nurse to educate the patient and family (caregiver) about the dying process, to keep them updated as the condition of the patient changes and to support the family during the last hours.[2]**

C. **The dying process is similar in chronic illness regardless of diagnosis. Hypoxia, malnutrition, hepatic and renal failure, fluid/electrolyte imbalance, and in cancer patients, tumor burden, gradually exhaust the body's coping mechanisms, resulting in death[3]**

II. **The Process of Dying—Goals of Care during the last days**

A. **Keep patient as comfortable as possible**

B. **Maintain the patient's sense of dignity**

C. **Avoid actions that might hasten death or prolong life**

D. **Prepare the family for the patient's final hours**

E.   **Re-evaluate plan of care based on changes in patient condition**

1.   Discontinue any medications that are no longer necessary, such as laxatives, hypoglycemics.

2.   Continue medications for pain, seizures, nausea

3.   Change oral medications to sublingual, rectal or, if necessary, to subcutaneous

III.   **Identification and Responses to Indicators of Imminent Death.**

A.   **There usually is a predictable set of processes that occur during the final stages of a terminal illness due to gradual hypoxia[4]**

B.   **Hypoxia does not manifest itself in signs and symptoms until the oxygen saturation drops below 80%**

C.   **At 65–80% oxygen saturation, the following signs and symptoms occur**

1.   Alteration in sensory perception, including impaired ability to grasp ideas and reason, periods of alertness along with periods of disorientation and restlessness

2.   Increased pulse and respiratory rate, periodic apnea, decreasing urinary output

3.   Some loss of visual acuity, increased sensitivity to bright lights; other senses, except hearing, are dulled

4.   Gradual increasing weakness beginning with the legs, then progressing to the arms and resulting in immobility

D.   **At 60% oxygen saturation and below, the following signs and symptom are present**

1.   Unresponsiveness

2.   Heart rate may double, strength of contractions decrease, rhythm becomes irregular; patient feels cool to the touch, and becomes diaphoretic; extremities may become mottled

3.   Eyes remain half open, blink reflex is absent; sense of hearing remains intact and slowly decreases

E.   **Predicting Time of Death**

1.   Morita, Ichiki, Tsunoda, Inoue, and Chihara[5], studied 4 common signs of impending death for onset and order of occurrence

2.   Death rattle preceded the other 3 symptoms in 74% of patients, and was first observed 24 hours or more prior to death in 49% of patients

3.   Respirations with mandibular movement followed, then cyanosis of extremities and pulselessness of the radial artery

4.   These last 3 symptoms were first observed during the final 6 hours in 68%, 81% and 87% of patients respectively; (The authors note that onset of symptoms and intervals to time of death varied individually, and death rattle did not occur in all patients)

IV. Terminal Symptoms

A. **Symptoms encountered in the last days of life vary in severity and occurrence**

1. The most common symptoms include noisy/moist breathing (death rattle), pain, urinary dysfunction, restlessness and agitation, and dyspnea[6]

2. These symptoms should be anticipated and a plan for management should be arranged prior to their occurrence if possible; (Note: Providing psychological/spiritual/existential support when appropriate is implied as part of the hospice/palliative philosophy of care)

B. **Altered Elimination**

1. Decreasing urinary output (can be sudden or gradual) is a normal part of the dying process related to shunting of blood supply away from the kidneys to the brain and heart

   a) Also consider: urinary retention; dehydration; ureteral obstruction

   b) Management options: treat underlying cause if appropriate; catheter, observation; reassure and teach regarding normal dying process

2. Urinary retention

   a) Inability to void, or inability to empty bladder completely

   b) May be caused by: tumor or nerve damage secondary to tumor, urethral stricture, spinal cord compression, drug side effects (especially anticholinergics), prostatic hypertrophy, fecal impaction, hematuria with blood clot retention, decreased level of consciousness[7]

   c) Management options: treat underlying cause if appropriate; disimpaction; medication changes; indwelling catheter

3. Incontinence—urinary

   a) Most often functional incontinence in the terminal phase due to cognitive impairment and profound weakness[3]

   b) Also consider: infection; tumor involvement, fecal impaction; medications (diuretics, alcohol, sedatives); atrophic vaginitis; fistula (usually seen as a continuous dribble of urine); urgency, bladder spasms

   c) Management options: treat underlying cause if appropriate; observation; reassure and teach regarding normal dying process; protective measures; absorbent pads/adult diapers, moisture barrier to perineum; indwelling catheter; teach regarding skin/catheter care

4. Fecal incontinence secondary to loss of sphincter control—may occur if diarrhea is present and patient is cognitively impaired

   a) Also consider: constipation; intestinal obstruction; distention; tenesmus; fecal impaction; steatorrhea; excessive laxative use; recto-vaginal fistula; medications (non-steroidal anti-inflammatory drugs [NSAIDs], antibiotics, antacids); spinal cord compression; chemotherapy; problems associated with enteral nutritional support

   b) Management options: treat underlying cause if appropriate; anti-diarrheal drugs, enzyme replacement, d/c or decrease enteral feeding (Sorbitol may be the offending ingredient)[8], observation; reassure and teach regarding normal dying process

C.   Altered breathing patterns

    1.   Cheyne-Stokes, periodic apnea

        a)   May be caused by: cerebral anoxia secondary to heart failure, aspiration or drug effects (especially in the opioid naive patient)

        b)   Management options: treat underlying cause if appropriate; oxygen if it adds comfort, observation; reassure and teach regarding normal dying process

    2.   Dyspnea

        a)   Treatment is the same in the terminal phase, regardless of cause[9]

        b)   Treatment options: morphine sulfate titrated to decrease respirations to 15–20/minute; lorazepam SL for accompanying anxiety; midazolam IV/SC for acute stridor; fan at bedside/cool environment with good ventilation; oxygen per nasal cannula in the presence of cyanosis or prn for comfort/psychological benefit; calm presence of loved ones; reassure and teach regarding dyspnea management and dying process

    3.   Respiratory congestion/death rattle: noisy, moist respirations, caused by the inability to clear pharyngeal and tracheal secretions, occur frequently prior to death. This symptom can be very distressing to caregivers, although the patient is probably not bothered by it

        a)   Also consider: congestive heart failure, over-hydration, neurological insult, pneumonia

        b)   Management options: treat underlying cause, if appropriate; oxygen for comfort, position on side in high fowler's position; anticholinergic medications (scopolamine, hyoscyamine) at the first sign of death rattle (will not dry up secretions already present; gentle oral suctioning may be necessary to clear accumulated secretions)[9] observation; reassure and teach regarding normal dying process

D.   Changes in mentation

    1.   Decreasing levels of consciousness, periods of lucidity, confusion, and nearing death transition

        a)   May be caused by: hypercalcemia, electrolyte imbalances, decreased blood glucose, increased ICP, cerebral metastasis, constipation, cerebral anoxia secondary to heart failure, drugs

        b)   Management options: treat underlying cause, if appropriate; d/c unnecessary drugs; haloperidol for marked confusion, chlorpromazine if sedation is desired; encourage family involvement; observation; reassure and teach regarding normal dying process

    2.   Restlessness and agitation (Refer to Chapter V)

        a)   Possible causes: pain, constipation, full bladder, dyspnea, paradoxical effect of sedatives, alcohol or benzodiazepine withdrawal, nausea, pruritis, anxiety and fear, unfinished business, congestion

        b)   Management options: treat underlying cause, if appropriate; use of sedatives (midazolam, chlorpromazine, haloperidol, barbiturates); consider opioid rotation and elimination of all medications that are not absolutely necessary; observation; reassure and teach regarding normal dying process[9, 10]

E. **Changes in reflex responses (Refer to Chapter V)**

  1. Dysphagia (difficult swallowing); odynophagia (pain on swallowing); impaired cough reflex

     a) May be caused by: candidiasis, mediastinal nodes, pharyngeal damage, neuromuscular changes as in ALS, fistula, local tumor recurrence of head and neck tumors, pervasive debilitation from multi-system decline, side effects of radiation or chemotherapy[11]

     b) Management options: treat underlying cause, if appropriate; positioning, change medication route to SL/topical/SC/PR; meticulous mouth care; determine food consistency best tolerated; use careful feeding techniques; observation; reassure and teach regarding prevention of aspiration and normal dying process

  2. Impaired corneal reflexes

     a) May be caused by: lack of humidity in room, dehydration

     b) Management options: treat underlying cause, if appropriate; artificial tears, eye care with cool cloths; humidity; observation; reassure and teach regarding normal dying process

F. **Circulatory changes**

  1. Edema (Refer to Chapter V)

     a) May be caused by: immobility, abdominal pressure, protein deficiency, lymphatic obstruction, deep vein thrombosis, inferior vena cava obstruction, heart failure

     b) Management options: treat underlying cause, if appropriate; passive range of motion (as tolerated early in the terminal phase); meticulous skin care aimed at prevention of skin breakdown; compression stockings, leg elevation, diuretics if edema is disturbing to the patient (combinations work best for stubborn edema); observation; reassure and teach regarding normal dying process

  2. Mottling, cyanosis, cool extremities

     a) Possible causes: drug effects, dehydration, internal bleeding, poor tissue perfusion secondary to heart failure

     b) Management options: treat underlying cause, if appropriate; position to minimize tissue damage and promote comfort; observation; reassure and teach regarding normal dying process

G. **Thermoregulatory changes**

  1. Hypothermia

     a) May be caused by: environmental temperature, poor tissue perfusion, decreased metabolic rate

     b) Management options: treat underlying cause, if appropriate; keep warm for comfort; observation; reassure and teach regarding normal dying process

2. Hyperthermia

    a) May be caused by: infection, tumor-induced fever, dehydration

    b) Management options: treat underlying cause, if appropriate; control fever for comfort with acetaminophen or NSAIDs, observation; reassure and teach regarding normal dying process

3. Diaphoresis

    a) Consider: infection, anxiety reactions, dyspnea, pain, malignant disease[12]

    b) Management options: treat underlying cause, if appropriate; steroids, indomethacin suppositories[3]; submersion in cool water, cool ambient temperatures, application of cool cloths[12]; observation; reassure and teach regarding normal dying process

H. Alteration in Comfort: Pain

1. May be caused by: disease progression, impaired absorption of opioids (especially when rectal medications are not placed against rectal mucosa), withholding of medication by caregiver, joint stiffness from immobility in the dying process

2. Management options: Continue previous opioid dosage unless there are signs of opioid toxicity; avoid abruptly discontinuing opioids (give at least 25% of previous dose to prevent withdrawal symptoms); minimize disturbance pain by premedicating prior to any procedure; gentle, slow repositioning; indomethacin suppositories for bone pain/joint stiffness; reassure and teach caregiver comfort measures, appropriate use of medications

V. Caregiver Support During the Final Days and Hours

A. Be reassuring and provide guidance as needed

1. Reassure caregivers of the interdisciplinary team's commitment to pain and symptom control. Rapid response to patient's changing needs and on-call availability demonstrate that commitment

2. Develop and teach crisis plan for anticipated distressing symptoms such as severe dyspnea or hemorrhage

3. Acknowledge the physical and emotional difficulties of providing end-of-life care, and affirm the value of caregiver's efforts and presence, regardless of the patient's responsiveness[9]

B. Prepare family/caregivers for what to expect as death approaches

1. Noisy or grunting respirations do not always mean that the dying person is in distress

2. Patient may still hear so be aware of what is said

3. Help family to contact others who are important to the patient and family

C. **Educate on signs and symptoms of approaching death and interventions to treat symptoms and minimize suffering.**

    1.   Inform family of disease progression

    2.   Teach the family that the patient may experience any number of the signs and symptoms described above or none

    3.   Intensive physical comfort care such as mouth care, turning and positioning

D. **Enhance and personalize a comfortable environment**

    1.   Prepare patient for any changes or disruptions

    2.   Avoid whispering

    3.   Provide consistency in caregivers

E. **Respect cultural, religious or spiritual rituals**

    1.   Be sensitive to patient and family needs

    2.   Ascertain significant rituals and activities; normalize appropriateness of silence, "being with", recognizing that patient may hear even when unable to respond

F. **Support family in honoring loved one's wishes to have a home or hospital death, DNR or resuscitation, and individualize care to support each person's values**

VI. **Signs that Death has Occurred**

A. **Lack of respirations**

B. **Lack of pulse**

C. **Incontinent of urine and stool**

D. **No verbal or nonverbal response**

E. **Eyelids may be slightly opened**

F. **Jaw relaxed and mouth slightly open**

VII. **Visit at Time of Death**

A. **Attendance at death provides support for patient and family—whether at home, in hospital or long term care facility; the task and focus will be determined by the place of death, and may include facilitating pronouncement, notification and transportation**

B.   Purposes for attendance include

1.   Provision of dignity, continuity, comfort and support for patient and family

2.   Confirmation that death has occurred, e.g., no breathing, pulse, pupillary reaction

3.   Notification of primary MD, hospice or palliative care team, coroner (depending upon local law), DME Company, mortuary or morgue as appropriate

4.   Opportunity for closure for hospice or palliative care staff member

C.   Tasks include

1.   Provision of comfort and support to patient and/or family at time of death

    a)   Allow for time alone with body, if desired

    b)   Honor cultural expectations

    c)   Assist with burial arrangements, when appropriate

2.   Facilitation of pronouncement of death (legal ability of RN to pronounce varies from state to state)

3.   Preparation of the body and bathing as needed; if appropriate, include family in carrying out this task

4.   Notification of appropriate persons/agencies

5.   Facilitation of rituals that may help family to integrate death and enhance coping or family closure and support

6.   Assistance to the mortuary at the time of removal of the body from the home, and when in the hospital preparation of the body for transportation to the morgue

7.   Assessment of family coping

    a)   Notify other team members for assistance as indicated

    b)   Deal with grief however it may be expressed

        (1)   Anger

        (2)   Sadness

        (3)   Guilt

        (4)   Apathy

        (5)   Hyperventilation

        (6)   Fainting

    c)   Reinforce continuing availability of staff and potential for bereavement services

REFERENCES

1. SUPPORT, S.P.I., *A controlled trial to improve care for seriously ill hospitalized patients: A study to understand prognoses and preferences for outcomes and risks of treatments (SUPPORT).* Journal of the American Medical Association, 1995. **274**: p. 1591–1598.

2. Matzo, M.L. and D.W. Sherman, *Palliative care nursing: Quality care to the end of life.* 2001, New York: Springer Publishing.

3. Enck, R., *The medical care of terminally ill patients.* 1994, Baltimore: Johns Hopkins University Press.

4. Kelly, C. and L. Yetman, *At the end of life.* Canadian Nurse, 1987. **83**(4): p. 33–34.

5. Morita, T., et al., *A prospective study on the dying process in terminally ill cancer patients.* The American Journal of Hospice and Palliative Care, 1987. **1**: p. 149–153.

6. Lichter, I. and E. Hunt, *The last 48 hours of life.* Journal of Palliative Care, 1990. **6**(4): p. 7–15.

7. Norman, R.W., *Genitourinary disorders, in Oxford Textbook of Palliative Medicine,* D. Doyle, G.W. Hanks, and N. MacDonald, Editors. 1998, Oxford University Press: New York. p. 667–676.

8. Sykes, N., *Constipation and diarrhea, in Oxford textbook of palliative medicine,* D. Doyle, G. Hanks, and N. MacDonald, Editors. 1998, Oxford: New York. p. 513–526.

9. Twycross, R. and I. Lichter, *The terminal phase, in Oxford Textbook of Palliative Medicine,* D. Doyle, G. Hanks, and N. MacDonald, Editors. 1998, Oxford University Press: New York. p. 977–992.

10. Kuebler, K.K., N. English, and D.E. Heidrich, *Delirium, confusion, agitation, and restlessness, in Textbook of Palliative Nursing,* B.R. Ferrell and N. Coyle, Editors. 2001, Oxford University Press: New York. p. 290–308.

11. Dahlin, C.M. and T. Goldsmith, *Dysphagia, dry mouth, & hiccups, in Textbook of Palliative Nursing,* B.R. Ferrell and N. Coyle, Editors. 2001, Oxford University Press: New York. p. 122–138.

12. Rhiner, M. and N.E. Slatkin, *Pruritis, fever, and sweats, in Textbook of Palliative Nursing,* B.R. Ferrell and N. Coyle, Editors. 2001, Oxford University Press: New York. p. 245–261.

GENERAL REFERENCES

Amenta, M.O. & Bohnet, N.L., (1986). *Nursing care of the terminally ill.* Boston: Little, Brown.

Berry, P. & Griffie, J. (2001). Planning for the actual death. In B.R. Ferrell & N. Coyle (Eds). *Textbook of Palliative Nursing.* New York, NY: Oxford University Press.

Callahan, M. & Kelley, P. (1993). *Final gifts: Understanding the special awareness, needs, and communications of the dying.* New York: Bantam Books.

Doyle, D., Hanks, G., & MacDonald, N. (Eds.). (1999). *Oxford textbook of palliative medicine.* (2nd Ed.) New York: Oxford University Press.

End-of-Life Nursing Education Consortium (ELNEC) (2001). Faculty Guide.

Emanuel, L.L, von Gunten, C.F., & Ferris, F.D. (1999). *The education for physicians on end-of-life education curriculum* (EPEC). www.EPEC.net: The EPEC Project.

Ferrell, B.R. & Coyle, N (Eds.). (2001). *Textbook of palliative nursing.* New York: Oxford University Press.

Hospice and Palliative Nurses Association. (2000). *Standards of hospice nursing practice and professional performance.* Pittsburgh: Author.

Johanson, G. (1994). *Physician handbook of symptom relief in terminal care* (4th ed.). Santa Rosa, CA: Sonoma County Academic Foundation for Excellence in Medicine, (1-707-527-6223).

Kemp, C. (1999). *Terminal illness: A guide to nursing care.* Philadelphia: J.B. Lippincott

Kuebler, K.K..(Ed.). (1997). *Hospice and palliative care clinical practice protocol: Terminal restlessness.* Dubuque: Kendall /Hunt Publishing Company.

Kuebler, K.K., Dahlin, C.M., Ladd, L., Montonye, M. & Zeri. K. (1996). *Hospice and palliative care clinical practice protocol: Dyspnea.* Pittsburgh: Hospice Nurses Association.

Larson, D. (1993). *The helper's journey: Working with people facing grief, loss, and life-threatening illness.* Champaign, IL: Research Press.

McIver, B. Walsh, D. & Nelson, K. (1994, July). The use of chlorpromazine for symptom control in dying cancer patients. *Journal of Pain and Symptom Management.* 9 (5): 341–345.

Johnston-Taylor, E. (1999). Caring for the spirit. In C.C. Burke (Ed). *Psychosocial dimensions of oncology nursing care.* Pittsburgh: Oncology Nursing Press.

Sheehan, D.C. & Forman, W.B. (1996). *Hospice and palliative care: Concepts and practice.* Boston: Jones & Bartlett.

Sheldon, J.E. (Ed.). (2000). *Hospice and palliative care clinical practice protocol: Nausea and vomiting.* Dubuque, IA: Kendall/Hunt Publishing.

Stoddard, S. (1991). *The hospice movement* (Rev. ed.). New York: Random House.

Volker, B.G. (Ed.). (1999). *Hospice and palliative nursing practice review.* (3rd ed.). Dubuque, IA: Kendall/Hunt Publishing.

Waller, A. & Caroline, N. (1996,) *Handbook of palliative care in cancer.* Boston: Butterworth-Heinemann.

Webb, M. (1997). *The good death: The new American search to reshaping the end of life.* New York: Bantam Books.

Wrede-Seaman, L. (1999). *Symptom management algorithms: A handbook for palliative care,* (2nd ed.). Yakima, WA: Intellicard.

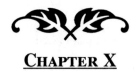

CHAPTER X

ECONOMIC ISSUES IN HOSPICE AND PALLIATIVE CARE

Barbara Volker, RN. MSN, CHPN
Ashby Watson, RN, MS, CS, OCN

I. **Economic Outcomes for End-of-Life Care**

    A. **Why measure economic outcomes?**

        1. To promote quality of care

        2. To control costs

        3. To benchmark for creative management

    B. **Economic issues affecting the provision of health care**

        1. Treatment costs and spending continue to rise

        2. High technology care is costly (1/2 of all Medicare spending occurs in the last six months of life)

        3. Increased consumer demand for sophisticated and expensive care

        4. Explosive growth of elderly population, who will survive longer with more chronic diseases

        5. Current insurance system rewards high technology interventions but does not reimburse for effective low technology interventions

    C. **Worldwide allocation of resources currently greatly favors curative care with less resources allocated to palliative care**

        1. World Health Organization (WHO) proposes[1]

            a) Greater allocation of palliative care resources to developing countries (survival not as great and palliative care needs are greater)

            b) More equal distribution of curative and comfort care resources in developed countries

D. Justification of Economic Outcomes[2]

1. Benefits should be weighed against toxicity and costs

2. Treatment justified if:

a) Improvement in overall survival

b) Improvement in disease-free survival

c) Improvement in quality of life

d) Improvement in cost effectiveness

e) Less toxicity occurs

3. Treatment should not be based on:

a) Cost alone

b) False hope that disease will improve or be cured

E. Economic evaluation of therapies for palliation

1. Hospice or Palliative Care may be a good economic choice[1]

a) Symptom relief

b) Prolongation of survival

c) If quality time is still available to the patient

2. Example: Chemotherapy for non-small cell lung cancer

a) Small benefit of 2–4 months survival[3]

b) May prevent hospitalizations late in disease course[2,4]

c) Benefit can be shown at reasonable cost[5,6]

F. The following factors also may influence cost outcomes

1. Less expensive the setting, the less costly the intervention

a) Home opioid infusions are less expensive than hospital infusions[7]

b) Outpatient chemotherapy is cheaper than inpatient chemotherapy[8]

c) Costs of home chemotherapy administration is less expensive than outpatient chemotherapy, making home chemotherapy a safe and economically realistic alternative to traditional hospital treatment[9]

d) Exception to this "rule" occurs in home health where IV medications may sometimes be given instead of oral because Medicare will pay for IV home infusion, but won't pay for oral medications

2. Care coordination[10,11]

a) Doesn't improve survival or symptom management outcomes, but can reduce costs by shortening hospital stays

b) Patient and family satisfaction increased[11,10]

3. Pain management coordination programs

    a) Reduction in admissions and re-admissions

    b) Can lead to marked cost savings[12]

4. Advanced Directives

    a) Research conflicting on cost-savings

        (1) No positive or negative impact on costs[13]

        (2) Patients who sign advance directive may have lower costs at last hospitalization [14]

        (3) If every person who died in 1988 executed an advance directive that was honored, selected hospice, refused aggressive in-hospital care, the total savings would have been $18.1 billion dollars (3.3% of all health care spending)[15]

    b) Barriers to completing Advance Directives[16]

        (1) People aren't always willing to sign advance directives

        (2) In the abstract, advance directives may be appealing, but when threat of death is real, people tend to opt for life-prolonging strategies

        (3) Health systems may not carry out patient's wishes anyway

        (4) If promoted as cost-saving strategy, public trust may be betrayed

        (5) Cultural issues

5. Ethics and Teaching Consultations[17]

    a) Surgical Intensive Care Unit (SICU) staff taught about dying and ethics of futile care

        (1) Reduced length of stay

        (2) SICU days significantly reduced

    b) Ethics consultations[18]

        (1) On all mechanically ventilated patients

        (2) Reduction in futile care

        (3) Increased transfers from ICU to lesser-intensity beds

        (4) Decreased costs because of less use of ICU

        (5) Ethics teaching and consultations

        (6) Palliative care consultations

II. **Access to Healthcare Systems at the End of Life**

    A. **Factors may vary from state to state**

        1. Scope of health care benefits limited

        2. Incentives for practitioners to provide less care

        3. Pre-authorization requirements

        4. Restricted eligibility

        5. Poor access of under-served populations

        6. Uninsured population, i.e., working poor, is growing

        7. Delayed referral to hospice and palliative care

        8. Cultural issues

    B. **Factors originating within the healthcare system**

        1. Patients discharged earlier and sicker

        2. Functionally disabled and cognitively impaired are increasingly admitted to long term care facilities

        3. Stress on ambulatory services and home care services to meet needs of growing populations

    C. **Financial impact**

        1. Medicare, Medicaid, Social Security are being pressured to cut costs

        2. Families taking on more of the burden:

            a) Lost work hours

            b) Out of pocket expenses

            c) Care hours by family members not reimbursed

            d) Caregiver stress and resultant poor health outcomes lead to increased use of health care system[16]

        3. Reported health care savings and costs may not reflect the actual cost of care for the full length of the illness

    D. **Potential cost savings in palliative care**

        1. Use of guidelines, algorithms, clinical pathways, flow sheets, standardized orders, and other disease management strategies

        2. Examples:

            a) HPNA Hospice and Palliative Care Clinical Practice Protocols/Monographs

            b) Algorithms for palliative care symptom management[19]

            c) NHPCO critical pathways for patients and families facing terminal illness

III. Reimbursement Sources for End-of-Life Care

    A.   **Common payor sources for end-of-life care in the United States[16]**

        1.   Medicare

        2.   Medicaid

        3.   Veterans and defense health programs

        4.   Employer sponsored programs

        5.   Private insurance plans

        6.   Uninsured

    B.   **Medicare is the most common source of payment for end-of-life care**

        1.   70% of those who die each year are elderly

        2.   13% of Medicare beneficiaries also receive Medicaid

        3.   28% of all Medicare payments is for care in the last year of life with nearly 50% of those costs incurred in the last 2 months of life[20]

        4.   For all beneficiaries, Medicare covered less than half of all health care expenses[21]

            a)   Medicaid paid 14%

            b)   Private insurance paid 10%

            c)   Family out of pocket expenses paid 10–20%[20]

            d)   Other resources paid 3%

        5.   Coverage limited for long term care, outpatient medications, supportive services

        6.   3/4 of beneficiaries have supplemental policies for medications, but those policies cover only 25% of prescription services (60% is paid out of pocket)

        7.   Those who qualify for Medicare hospice benefit may receive some medications and non-medical services

        8.   Hospice accounts for 1% of Medicare spending, 1/10 of 1% of Medicaid spending[22]

        9.   Medicare expenditures influences:

            a)   Costs at end of life may be a function of population growth, general economic inflation, and additional medical inflation[16]

            b)   National Medical Care Expenditure Survey[23] found that in the last year of life of those who died in 1988:

                (1)   For those younger than 65, costs of 44.9 billion were 7.5% of total health care expenditures

                (2)   For those older than 65, costs of $32.6 billion were 5.5% of total health care expenditures

            c)   Time to death—more money spent in year prior to death

            d)   Cause of death—payments influenced by disease and its treatment

e)   Age at death—payments per decedents dropped the older the person was at death, but those who survived may have had more chronic illnesses, thus increasing costs

f)   Cost offsets—for those persons who had both Medicare and Medicaid, lower Medicare costs may be offset by higher Medicaid costs

g)   Family costs—families may be assuming a larger part of the financial responsibility for care

C.   **Medicare hospice reimbursement via the Medicare Hospice Benefit**[24]

1.   Under Medicare Part A (is seen as an alternative to hospitalization)

2.   Patient must be Medicare eligible

3.   Electing the hospice Medicare benefit requires that the patient give informed consent. If the patient lacks decision-making capacity, a surrogate decision-maker may give the informed consent

a)   Essential elements of an informed consent for hospice admission; patient/surrogate must be informed of:

(1)   Palliative nature of services, and definition of the services

(2)   Service settings, home care, acute inpatient care, respite, residential settings

(3)   Bereavement services

(4)   Services covered and not covered

(5)   Financial responsibility

(6)   Withdrawal or discharge criteria

b)   If the patient has capacity to make health care decisions, he/she must sign the consent form

c)   In any situation where the patient does not sign the consent and or benefit election form, the reason must be clearly documented

4.   Terminally ill with less than 6 month prognosis (if the disease runs its usual course)

5.   Prognosis certified by primary MD and hospice medical director for first benefit period; by hospice medical director for subsequent benefit periods

6.   The scope of service is defined as palliative treatment related to the terminal illness

7.   Benefit periods

a)   There are two 90 day benefit periods and unlimited 60 day periods, as long as the patient remains appropriate for hospice care[25]

b)   Patients may sign off of, or **revoke**, the Medicare hospice benefit and resume traditional Medicare coverage for the terminal illness. Any remaining days in that benefit period are forfeited.

8. **Important note:** the Medicare hospice regulations *apply to the care of all patients* in a Medicare certified hospice

    a)   Except for the 80/20 rule (see below) and requirement that the hospice continue to provide services regardless of ability to pay or bill a third party payer

    b)   **Therefore, Medicare defines the delivery of hospice care in the U.S.**

9. **"Core services"** is a term used by Medicare to designate those team members that must be provided by the agency and not arranged for by contract (nurses, medical social services, and counseling); this in no way negates the requirement for a more comprehensive team; other team members may be employees of the agency or their services may be arranged by contract

10. Must also provide therapy services (PT, OT, speech-language pathology), physician, volunteer, home health aide and homemaker services, medical supplies and equipment; acute and respite inpatient care, medications related to terminal illness, bereavement services; can be provided under contract

11. Levels of care in Medicare hospice program

    a)   **Routine home care day:** A day in which a hospice patient receives care at home and is not receiving continuous care

    b)   **Continuous home care day:** A day in which a hospice patient receives care at home for brief periods of crisis necessary to maintain the patient at home

        (1)   Continuous care is furnished during brief periods of crisis and only as necessary to maintain the terminally ill patient at home

        (2)   Care is provided for at least 8 hours a day in order to qualify for the continuous home care reimbursement rate (Medicare defines the "day" as one that starts and ends at midnight)

        (3)   Care must consist of predominantly (more than 50%) skilled nursing care (RN or LPN/LVN)

    c)   **Inpatient respite care:** A day in which a hospice patient receives care in an approved facility on a short-term basis for respite of family or other caregivers

        (1)   The hospice will not be reimbursed for respite care more than 5 days consecutively

        (2)   Payment to the hospice program for the sixth and any subsequent day of respite care is made at the routine home care rate

    d)   **General inpatient care:** A day in which a hospice patient receives care in an approved facility for pain control or symptom management when care is not feasible in other settings (home or continuous care)

        (1)   Inpatient caps

            (a)   Medicare has established a limit to the number of total patient care days that will be reimbursed at either the general inpatient or inpatient respite care rates

            (b)   The total inpatient days for Medicare patients may not exceed 20% of the total days for all those patients who elect the Medicare hospice benefit in any Medicare fiscal year (this is sometimes described as the 80/20 rule)

e) **Change in level of care within the Medicare Hospice benefit**

    (1)   Transfer to another level of care is based on the medical needs of the patient (e.g. uncontrolled pain)

    (2)   Change in level of care requires a discussion with the patient and family, and the IDT, changes in the plan of care, the primary physician's order, documentation in the patient's record

12. Volunteer Services

   a)   Volunteer service hours must account for 5% of all direct patient care hours for all paid hospice employees and contract staff in a Medicare certified hospice program

   b)   The volunteer hours may be accumulated as direct patient care hours or indirect, administrative support hours

13. Issues associated with the *discontinuation* of hospice care (other than by death of the patient and the completion of the bereavement period for the family):

   a)   Patient/family initiated actions

    (1)   **Transfer:** hospice care is transferred when a patient moves out of the service area of one hospice and into another hospice's service area or chooses a different provider in the area: patient remains in the current benefit period and loses no days in that period

       (a)   Role of the hospice in facilitating patient transfer to a different care setting is to:

          (i)   Coordinate with the other hospice/palliative care service in order to provide continuity of care

          (ii)   Notify the physician of the change in service area and/or service provider

       (b)   Hospice Medicare/Medicaid benefit patients may transfer only once per benefit period

    (2)   **Withdrawal:** any patient/family can choose to discontinue all services of the hospice for any reason.

       (a)   Role of the hospice in facilitating patient/family withdrawal from service

          (i)   Notify primary physician of change and initiate any paperwork necessary for the change

          (ii)   Coordinate any referrals for provision of on-going medical care

       (b)   The choice to withdraw from hospice care requires the patient/legal representative to **revoke** the hospice benefit

(3) **Revocation** of the Medicare Hospice Benefit is an option that may be chosen by the patient/family in order to receive treatment not covered under the hospice plan of care, to receive care from a different service provider, e.g. skilled nursing facility, non-contracted hospital, or because of dissatisfaction with the service being provided

    (a) **Revocation:** may occur any time during a benefit period; a patient may choose to revoke his/her Medicare hospice (note: the hospice program may not instruct the patient and family to revoke)

    (b) Notify the physician of the change from hospice

    (c) Have patient sign the Revocation statement/form on the date he/she revoked

    (d) Be sure to indicate the date and time the form was signed

b) Hospice program initiated actions

(1) **Discharge:** a patient who no longer meets the Medicare criteria may be discharged; otherwise, this action is only used in extraordinary circumstances.

    (a) Example: a patient may be discharged if continuing to provide care poses a serious threat to the safety of staff

    (b) A patient MAY NOT be discharged because of inability to pay for services, if the management of the illness and palliative treatment is too expensive for the hospice, if the primary physician orders expensive, "high tech" palliative care, or if they are "difficult" to care for

(2) **Non-recertification:** (also referred to as "decertification") At the end of a benefit period, the hospice Interdisciplinary Team, with the patient's primary physician, determines the patient no longer has a prognosis of 6 months or less (if the disease runs its normal course); a change in the status of the patient's terminal condition is the ONLY consideration justifying non-recertification

c) Role of the hospice program in discontinuation of care; the hospice program is responsible to:

(1) Notify the patient and family of the reasons for discontinuation of services

(2) Inform the patient and family that the hospice benefit is still available to them if the need arises later

(3) Provide for continuity of care when transferring patient and family care to another agency

14. Actual and potential problems inherent in the Medicare Hospice Benefit

a) Medicare Hospice Benefit criteria may cause delayed hospice referrals, limiting access to care

(1) Trend in decline of length of stay for hospice

(2) Imminent death is primary stimulus for hospice referral

(3) 9% of patients die before they can be admitted to hospice even when admitted 24 hours from time of referral[26, 27]

      (4)   Crisis care mode with emphasis on just getting pain and symptoms under control

      (5)   Rarely time for hospice team to form therapeutic relationships with families

b)   Effective palliative care efforts so close to death may increase costs and negatively impact on quality of care

c)   Expenses for patients who desire costly life-prolonging treatment may negatively impact hospice's bottom line

d)   Current hospice *per diem* reimbursement has the potential to result in negative outcomes:

      (1)   Could discourage the use of effective, but more costly pain medications even when less expensive drugs fail[28, 29]

      (2)   Might discourage nursing visits (especially after hours) to help families in crisis

      (3)   Might discourage the appropriate application of high-tech equipment

      (4)   Might discourage extensive counseling that may be useful for particularly distressed patients

e)   Increased family costs—data have begun to indicate that families are shouldering not only the physical burden of care, but an increasingly larger portion of the financial burden[1]

f)   Requirement for primary caregiver may deny access to hospice or cause financial hardship

      (1)   75% of single-parent households headed by women who work[30]

      (2)   To access benefit[31] a caregiver may have to:

          (a)   Take leave of absence

          (b)   Use family medical leave (12 weeks without pay)

          (c)   Quit job

g)   Residents and families of residents in skilled nursing facilities who are appropriate both for the Medicare hospice benefit and for Medicare skilled care days may be negatively impacted

      (1)   Because it is to the economic advantage of the skilled nursing facility to have the resident on Medicare skilled care days, facility staff may not fully inform resident and family of their right to receive hospice care

      (2)   A resident and family who chose hospice care instead of Medicare skilled days must bear the economic burden of paying room and board for the resident because Medicare does not provide that as part of the hospice benefit

D.   Medicaid reimbursement under the Medicaid Hospice Benefit

1.   In most states with a Medicaid hospice benefit the hospice benefit and reimbursement for care is modeled after the Medicare Hospice Benefit

   a)   The hospice nurse is responsible for knowing any differences between the Medicare hospice benefit and the Medicaid benefit as it is established in the geographical area served by the hospice

   b)   This is especially important to keep in mind if the hospice serves more than one state

2.   Actual and potential problems inherent in the Medicaid Hospice Benefit

   a)   Hospice is an optional benefit under the Medicaid program and not all states chose to provide it

   b)   Because of the similarity between the Medicare and Medicaid hospice benefits most of the other actual or potential problems are the same as well (see Section III B #14)

E.   Reimbursement for palliative care under Medicare

1.   No formal reimbursement system for palliative care therapies exists[32]

2.   Palliative Care DRG[33]

   a)   DRG codes are used by Health Care Financing Administration to define how Medicare funds are reimbursed

   b)   Reimbursement for palliative care is limited

   c)   In 1996 an ICD-9-CM "v66.7" code for palliative care was developed; does not actually bring reimbursement, but allows data to be collected about the provision of palliative care services

      (1)   To determine if new code is needed to pay hospitals

      (2)   To determine if it is feasible to reimburse for palliative care

3.   Demonstration projects and innovative programs developed to integrate palliative care approaches and to improve quality of end of life care

   a)   Robert Wood Johnson Initiative on Improving Care at the End of Life

   b)   Project ENABLE

   c)   Wisconsin Resource Manual for Improvement

   d)   City of Hope Pain Resource Center

   e)   The Institute for Healthcare Improvement Collaborative

   f)   United Hospital Fund's Hospital Palliative Care Initiative

   g)   Veterans Health Administration 5th Vital Sign program

F. Reimbursement for hospice and palliative care under private insurance benefit plans

1. Hospice reimbursement under private insurance benefit plans

    a) About 80 % of private insurance plans have a hospice benefit; most others will negotiate a rate for hospice; some use a home health benefit

        (1) Many hospices refuse to "unbundle" hospice services even when insurance companies only pay for some aspects of the program

        (2) If a program is Medicare certified, all patients must receive all the services available to a Medicare beneficiary whether or not the insurance company pays

    b) Types of plans

        (1) **Per Diem**—reimbursement to the hospice is similar to Medicare/Medicaid in that it is on a daily basis and includes all services

        (2) **Per visit**—insurance company authorizes the number of visits and the disciplines visiting

            (a) Services not involving visits such as bereavement and participation in interdisciplinary team meetings are not reimbursed

            (b) The insurance company may not authorize other services such as spiritual counseling

            (c) Many hospices will not accept per visit reimbursement

        (3) **Dollar caps**—the patient has a benefit with a limited amount of money; for example, $5,000 lifetime maximum per patient for hospice

            (a) The hospice may be at financial risk if the cost of care exceeds the cap

            (b) Many hospices continue the care when the cap is exceeded and provide services without compensation

        (4) **Negotiated rates**—rate of reimbursement is individualized according to the plan of care and agreement reached between the hospice and the insurance provider

2. Palliative care reimbursement under private insurance benefit plans

    a) Palliative care services (non-hospice benefits) generally are reimbursable under various parts of the patient's medical insurance, e.g. hospital medical services, physician medical services, etc. (part of the specialty consult process):

        (1) Determined by the IDT to be necessary

        (2) Follow agency/provider guidelines and reimbursement requirements for obtaining medications, medical equipment, and supplies

3. Actual and potential problems inherent in the provision of care under private insurance

    a) Availability and type of insurance affect the use and provision of health care[34, 35, 36, 37]

    b) Managed health care plans have limited scopes and levels of benefits

        (1) Use can ease the financial burden of illness and encourage people to obtain beneficial care[38]

(2)   Utilization increases costs, so insurance companies use a variety of means to discourage use of their resources

c)   Uninsured patients

(1)   Cannot be turned away if they have acute or life-threatening problems[16]

(2)   Care paid for by special public or charitable funds, application for public insurance

d)   Penalizes those with advanced disease[38]

e)   Bias risk selection—purpose is to attract healthy participants, not sick ones

(1)   Exclude pre-existing conditions

(2)   The sicker one is, the more one has to pay out of pocket for care

(3)   Additional caps

(a)   Outpatient prescription medications excluded

(b)   Deductibles, coinsurance payments

(c)   Caps on visits or days of care, dollar amounts of payments, defined time periods

(d)   No upper limits on beneficiary liability for cost-sharing

f)   Financial Incentives for clinicians to provide less care[38]

(1)   Fixed payments per day, per case, per capita

(2)   Plans may vary in capitation of services

(3)   Pre-authorization requirements

(a)   Require approval prior to obtaining service

(b)   "Gatekeepers" to approve specialist visits

(4)   Protocols developed by the insurance companies require:

(a)   Specific services to be given for certain diseases

(b)   Specific medications from designated formularies

(5)   Productivity standards for physician appointments

(a)   Visits may be limited by plan expectations

(b)   Impact may be less time spent with patients

(6)   Health plan "panel" limitations

(a)   Patient may use only designated physicians

(b)   Out-of-plan costs are greater

(c)   Limitations on specialized services such as pain management specialists

(d)   Both access and length of time to appointment can be affected

(e)   Frequent denials from insurance companies due to lack of knowledge about palliative care and/or equating it with hospice care

IV. Relevant Economic Issues in End-of-Life Care

A. In the hospital setting

1. DRG prospective payment system[38]

2. Assumes that hospitals get a mix of patients so costs can be averaged out over all patients

a) Hospital stays are paid on a prospectively determined, diagnosis-related basis

b) If hospitals can discharge patients ahead of time, they get to keep any money they've made

c) Outlier patients are high cost patients; hospital costs for these patients must reach certain designated levels before the hospital is reimbursed

3. Actual or potential effect of the prospective payment system on end-of-life care in the hospital setting:

a) Shorter hospital stays have not been offset by increased admissions

b) Shorter stays have put increased burden on the family

(1) Drug costs

(2) Huge burden on those with dying family members

c) Early studies showed early discharge, but no negative impact on mortality[39, 40, 41, 42, 43]

d) Premature discharge from hospital may leave families without adequate support systems to manage care

(1) Home care system not in place or inadequate

(2) Symptom management expertise may vary

(3) Hospice coverage for inpatient care is limited

e) Issues for palliative care in the hospital setting

(1) How to identify homogeneous care resources (not tied to diagnosis) that can be reimbursed and monitored

(2) Not intended to discourage referral to hospice

(3) No data yet released on the palliative care ICD-9 code

B. Issues for physicians who care for the dying

1. Importance of coding visits for "evaluation and management" vs. procedures and tests

2. Different codes exist for brief, limited, extended and other classes

3. Codes do not differentiate between classes of patients[44, 45]

a) May discourage care of those with special needs

(1) Hearing/sight/cognitively impaired

(2) Those requiring special symptom management

(3) Those with needs for emotional support

b) Restrictive interpretation of codes may limit physician time spent with these patients[16]

  4. Nursing home visits not reimbursed at same level as hospital visits

C. **Issues in the skilled nursing facility where most funding comes from Medicaid**

  1. 7 of 10 residents receive some funding from Medicaid[46]

  2. 12% of beneficiaries accounted for 33% of total expenditures, much accounted for by nursing home use[47]

  3. Not all states adjust payments based on nursing home case mix[48]

    a) Discourages nursing homes from accepting sicker patients

    b) Discourages nursing homes from providing adequate level of care

  4. Nursing home populations are more severely ill and impaired and more demanding of resources due to:

    a) Reduced hospital lengths of stay

    b) More sophisticated technological care; nursing home staff are not usually able to provide such care; systems not in place

    c) Increasing resident age and disability

  5. Recent data on Medicare hospice care in skilled nursing facilities in five states from 1992 to 1996[49] demonstrated:

    a) Hospice care is associated with less hospitalization for Medicare hospice patients

    b) Diffusion of palliative care philosophy and practices to care of non-hospice residents resulted in lower rates of end-of-life hospitalizations as well.

D. **Provision of hospice services**

  1. Hospice benefit was originally adopted after years of increased Medicare spending[16]; it was designed to control costs

    a) Limit number of qualifying beneficiaries (6 month life expectancy)

    b) Encourage efficient and economical home care

      (1) Four levels of per diem payment rates

      (2) Overall cap on payments

    c) Discourage inpatient care with per diem payment for inpatient care and 20% cap on aggregate hospital payments

    d) Required use of volunteers limits Medicare liability for some care

  2. Capitation of hospice is characterized by many as "high-risk"[16]

    a) Lack of data on incidence and variability of terminal illness

    b) Variability across populations

      (1) Lack of effective tools to detect and deflect inappropriate early referrals to hospice

      (2) Lack of other information needed to set rates and manage financial risk

3.   Medicare HMO beneficiaries' election of hospice benefit

  a)   Not limited only to HMO-selected hospice

  b)   HMO's not required to provide hospice benefits themselves

  c)   HMO's cannot deny access to HCFA-certified hospice

4.   Hospice coverage for those not eligible for Medicare or Medicaid varies greatly—80% of large and medium-size companies offer hospice coverage[50]

E.   **Issues for Home Health Care in providing palliative care services**

  1.   Eligibility requirements:

    a)   Patient must be homebound

    b)   Patient must need part-time or intermittent skilled nursing care or physical or speech therapy

  2.   Growth in home care expenditures[51]

    a)   Changes in Medicare home care policies

    b)   Growing supply of providers

    c)   Earlier discharge from hospitals

    d)   Increased feasibility of providing advanced technology in the home

  3.   Demonstration projects currently examining quality of care, efficiency, and cost control due to past evidence of fraud and abuse[52]

  4.   Cost shifting in home care has been documented[53]

    a)   Savings from averted hospital care may be offset by increased financial burden on family

    b)   Clauser reported that Medicare home care users were more likely to be disabled, living alone, poor and receiving Medicaid when compared to nonusers[16]

  5.   Medication coverage issues in palliative home care pose significant problems for patients and families[54, 29]

    a)   Medicare home care benefit does not cover medications in most cases

      (1)   Some supplemental policies cover outpatient prescriptions (programs vary)

      (2)   Some cover prescriptions but limit refills, number of prescriptions covered in a month, or quantity of medication

    b)   Examples of inefficiency:

      (1)   Oral medications and transdermal patches are not covered for outpatients[29]

      (2)   Use of infusion pump if not indicated, a more expensive option and one that may cause more complications, can be used in home, e.g., compare costs of $4,000 pump versus $100 for oral medication however may be essential for pain management in some patient's pain

F.   Economic value of the Advanced Practice Nurse (APN) in hospice and palliative care settings

1.   APN definitions:

a)   Application of an expanded range of practical, theoretical, and research-based therapeutics to phenomena experienced by patients within a specialized clinical area of the larger discipline of nursing

b)   Advanced practice registered nurses manifest a high level of expertise in the assessment, diagnosis, and treatment of the complex responses of individuals, families, or communities to actual or potential health problems, prevention of illness and injury, maintenance of wellness, and provision of comfort[55]

c)   The advanced practice registered nurse has a master's or doctoral education concentrating in a specific area of advanced nursing practice, had supervised practice during graduate education, and has ongoing clinical experiences[55]

d)   Advanced practice registered nurses continue to perform many of the same interventions used in basic nursing practice; the difference in this practice relates to a greater depth and breadth of knowledge, a greater degree of synthesis of data, and complexity of skills and interventions[55]

2.   Practice Models

a)   Should provide clarity and direction to the field

b)   Purposes served are determined by the concepts delineated in the framework, i.e., practice competencies

c)   Competency is core concept in several APN practice models:

(1)   Model of Expert Practice[56, 57]

(2)   Expert Practice Domains of the CNS and NP[58,59]

(3)   Model of Advanced Nursing Practice[60]

(4)   Model of Nurse Practitioner Practice[61]

3.   Factors indicating a need for advanced practice nurses who specialize in end of life care

a)   British nurses specializing in palliative care have raised the general standard of care and increased patient satisfaction

b)   Our evolving health care system places more emphasis on integration of care across different settings and over a continuum of life

c)   Studies increasingly are demonstrating the APN role can improve quality of life in a cost-effective way[62, 63, 64]

4. As a member of the interdisciplinary palliative care team, the Advanced Practice Nurse assumes many roles as he/she interfaces with families, staff, colleagues, and communities[65]

    a) Advanced clinician

    b) Educator

    c) Researcher

    d) Consultant

    e) Role Model

    f) Mentor

5. Advanced practice nurses who specialize in end of life care should be:

    a) Resourceful and flexible in interactions with dying patients and families

    b) Accepting of a broadened definition of palliative care that includes earlier service to a population with life-threatening illness

    c) Comfortable with technologies that employ both drug and non-drug technologies for pain and symptom control

    d) Advocates for patient and family self-determination

    e) Able to accommodate and advocate for family needs while negotiating with multiple health care professionals in a variety of settings

REFERENCES

1. Coyne, P., L. Lyckholm, and T.J. Smith, *Clinical interventions, economic outcomes, and palliative care,* in *Textbook of palliative nursing,* B. Ferrell and N. Coyle, Editors. 2001, Oxford University Press: New York.

2. American Society of Clinical Oncology Outcomes Working Group (ASCO), c.m., *Outcomes of cancer treatment for technology assessment and cancer treatment guidelines.* Journal of Clinical Oncology, 1995. **14:** p. 671–679.

3. Souquet, P.J., et al., *Polychemotherapy in advanced non-small cell lung cancer: A meta-analysis.* Lancet, 1993. **342:** p. 19–21.

4. Jaakkimainen, L., et al., *Counting the costs of chemotherapy in a National Cancer Institute of Canada randomized trial in non-small cell lung cancer.* Journal of Clinical Oncology, 1990. **8**(8): p.1301–1309.

5. LeChavlier, T., et al., *Randomized study of vinorelbine and cisplatin versus vindesine and cisplatin versus vinorelbine alone in advanced non-small cell lung cancer: results of a European multicenter trial including 612 patients.* Journal of Clinical Oncology, 1994. **12**(2): p. 360–367.

6. Smith, T.J., et al., *An economic evaluation of a randomized clinical trial comparing vinorelbine, vinorelbine plus cisplatin and vindesine plus cisplatin for non-small cell lung cancer.* Journal of Clinical Oncology, 1995. **13**(9): p. 6–2173.

7. Ferris, F.D., et al., *A cost-minimization study of cancer patients requiring a narcotic infusion in hospice and at home.* Journal of Clinical Epidemiology, 1991. **44**(3): p. 313–327.

8. Wodinsky, H.B., et al., *Re-evaluating the cost of outpatient cancer chemotherapy.* Canadian Medical Association Journal, 1987. **137**(10): p. 903–906.

9. Lowenthal, R.M., et al., *Home chemotherapy for cancer patients: Cost analysis and safety.* Medical Journal of Australia, 1996. **165**(4): p. 184–187.

10. Addington-Hall, J.M., L.D. MacDonald, and H.R. Anderson, *Randomized controlled trial of effects of coordinating care for terminally ill patients.* British Medical Journal, 1992. **305:** p. 1317–1322.

11. Raftery, J.P., et al., *A randomized controlled trial of the cost-effectiveness of a district co-coordinating service for terminally ill cancer patients.* Palliative Medicine, 1996. **10:** p. 151–161.

12. Grant, M., et al., *Unscheduled readmissions for uncontrolled symptoms.* Nursing Clinics of North America, 1995. **30:** p. 673–682.

13. SUPPORT, S.P.I., *A controlled trial to improve care for seriously ill hospitalized patients: A study to understand prognoses and preferences for outcomes and risks of treatments (SUPPORT).* Journal of the American Medical Association, 1995. **274:** p. 1591–1598.

14. Weeks, W.B., et al., *Advance directives and the cost of terminal hospitalization.* Archives of Internal Medicine, 1994. **154**(18): p. 2077–2083.

15. Emanuel, E.J. and L. Emanuel, *The economics of dying: The illusion of cost savings at the end of life.* New England Journal of Medicine, 1994. **330**(8): p. 540–544.

16. Field, M.J. and C.K. Cassel, *Approaching death: Improving care at the end of life.* 1997, Institute of Medicine Task Force: Washington, DC.

17. Holloran, S.D., et al., *An educational intervention in the surgical intensive care unit to improve ethical decisions.* Surgery, 1995. **118**(2): p. 294–298.

18. Dowdy, M.D., C. Robertson, and J.A. Bander, *A study of proactive ethics consultation for critically and terminally ill patients with extended lengths of stay.* Critical Care Medicine, 1998. **26**(2): p.252–259.

19. Wrede-Seaman, L., *Symptom management algorithms: A handbook for palliative care.* 2nd Edition ed. 1999, Yakima, WA: Intellicard.

20. National Hospice and Palliative Care Organization, *Facts and figures on hospice care in America.* 2001, National Hospice and Palliative Care Organization.

21. Gornick, M., A. McMillan, and J.A. Lubitz, *A longitudinal perspective on patterns of medicare payments.* Health Affairs, 1996. **12**(2): p. 140–150.

22. National Hospice Organization, *Hospice fact sheet.* 1996, National Hospice Organization: Arlington.

23. Cohen, S.B., B.L. Carlson, and D.E.B. Potter, *Health care expenditures in the last six months of life.* Health Policy Review, 1995. **1**(2): p. 1–13.

24. Health Care Financing Administration (HCFA), *Transmittal #256: Medicare state operations manual.* 1994, (HCFA): Baltimore. p. Sections 2080–2087.

25. *Balanced Budget Act,* in Congressional Record. 1997. p. Chapter 5.

26. Jackson, A., *Oregon hospice statistics and trends (draft 3/3/98).* 1998, Oregon Hospice Association: Portland.

27. Oregon Hospice Association, *Hospice in Oregon—a profile.* 1998, Oregon Hospice Association: Portland.

28. Brown, G., *Statement before the IOM Committee on Care at the End of Life on behalf of Hospice of the Blue Grass,* in *IOM Committee on Care at the End of Life.* 1996: Washington, DC.

29. Joranson, D.E., *Are health-care reimbursement policies a barrier to acute and cancer pain management?* Journal of Pain and Symptom Management, 1994. **9**(4): p. 244–253.

30. Emanuel, E.J., et al., *Assistance from family members, friends, paid care givers, and volunteers in the care of terminally ill patients.* New England Journal of Medicine, 1999. **341**(13): p. 956–63.

31. Covinsky, K.E., et al., *The impact of serious illness on patients' families. SUPPORT Investigators. Study to understand prognoses and preferences for outcomes and risks of treatment.* Journal of the American Medical Association, 1994. **272**: p. 1839–1844.

32. Whedon, M.B., *Hospital care, in Textbook of palliative nursing,* B. Ferrell and N. Coyle, Editors. 2001, Oxford University Press: New York.

33. Cassel, C., *Letter to colleagues about new Medicare palliative care code.* 1996, Milbank Memorial Fund: New York.

34. Hadley, J., E.P. Steinberg, and J. Feder, *Comparison of uninsured and privately insured hospital patients: Condition on admission, resource use, and outcome.* Journal of the American Medical Association, 1991. **265**(3): p. 274–279.

35. Manning, W.G., et al., *Health insurance and the demand for medical care: Evidence from a randomized experiment.* American Economic Review, 1987. **77**(3): p. 251–277.

36. Braveman, P., et al., *Adverse outcomes and lack of health insurance among newborns in an eight-county area of California.* New England Journal of Medicine, 1998. **321**: p. 508–513.

37. Newhouse, J.P. and I.E. Group, *Free for all? Lessons from the Rand Health Insurance Experiment.* 1993, Harvard University Press: Cambridge.

38. Millman, M., *Access to health care in America.* 1993, Institute of Medicine—National Academy Press: Washington, DC.

39. ProPAC, P.P.A.C., *Medicare and the American health care system: Report to the congress.* 1985, ProPac: Washington, DC.

40. ProPAC, P.P.A.C., *Medicare and the American health care system: Report to the congress.* 1989, ProPac: Washington, DC.

41. Kahn, K.L., et al., *Comparing outcomes of care before and after implementation of the DRG-based prospective payment system.* Journal of the American Medical Association, 1990. **264**(15): p.1984–1988.

42. Kosecoff, J., et al., *Prospective payment system and impairment at discharge.* Journal of the American Medical Association, 1990. **264**(15): p. 1980–1983.

43. Rubenstein, L.B., et al., *Changes in quality of care for five diseases measured by implicit review, 1981–1986.* Journal of the American Medical Association, 1990. **264**(15): p. 1974–1979.

44. PPRC, P.P.R.C., *Annual report to congress.* 1991, PPRC: Washington, DC.

45. PPRC, P.P.R.C., *Annual report to congress.* 1992, PPRC: Washington, DC.

46. American Health Care Association, A., *Facts and trends: The nursing facility sourcebook.* 1995, American Health Care Association, (AHCA): Washington, DC.

47. PPRC, P.P.R.C., *Annual report to congress.* 1993, PPRC, Physician Payment Review Commission: Washington, DC.

48. Swan, J.H., S. Dewit, and C. Harrington, *State Medicaid reimbursement methods and rates for nursing homes,* 1993. 1994, Wichita State University: Wichita, KS.

49. Miller, S.C., P. Gozalo, and V. Mor, *Hospice enrollment and hospitalization of dying nursing home patients.* American Journal of Medicine, 2001. **111**(1): p. 38–44.

50. Snow, C., *New hospice horizons: HMO expansion could boost providers popularity.* Modern Healthcare, 1997. **27**(9): p. 90, 92.

51. Health Care Financing Administration (HCFA), *Trends in Medicare home health agency utilization and payment: Cys 1974-94.* Health Care Financing Review, 1996. **Statistical Suppl**: p. 76–77.

52. Clauser, S.B., *Recent innovations in home health care policy research.* Health Care Financing Review, 1994. **16**(1): p. 1–6.

53. Weissert, W.G., *A new policy agenda for home care.* Health Affairs, 1991. **10**(2): p. 67–77.

54. Sourmerasi, S.B., et al., *Effects of Medicaid drug-payment limits on admission to hospitals and nursing homes.* New England Journal of Medicine, 1987. **325**(15): p. 1072–1077.

55. American Nurses Association, *Scope and standards of advanced practice registered nursing.* 1996, Washington, DC: American Nurses Association.

56. Benner, P., *From novice to expert.* 1984, Menlo Park: Addison-Wesley.

57. Benner, P., *The oncology clinical nurse specialist as expert coach.* Oncology Nursing Forum, 1985. **12**(2): p. 40–44.

58. Fenton, M.V., *Identifying competencies of clinical nurse specialists.* Journal of Nursing Administration, 1985. **15**(12): p. 31–37.

59. Fenton, M.V. and K.A. Brykczynski, *Qualitative distinctions and similarities in the practice of clinical nurse specialists and nurse practitioners.* Journal of Professional Nursing, 1993. **9**: p.313–326.

60. Calkin, J.D., *A model for advanced nursing practice*. Journal of Nursing Administration, 1984. **14**(1): p. 24–30.

61. Shuler, P.A. and J.E. Davis, *The Shuler nurse practitioner practice model: A theoretical framework for nurse practitioner clinicians, educators, and researchers. Part I*. Journal of the American Academy of Nurse Practitioners, 1993. **5**: p. 11–18.

62. Rich, M., et al., *A multidisciplinary intervention to prevent the readmission of elderly patients with congestive heart failure*. The New England Journal of Medicine, 1995. **333**(18): p. 1190–1195.

63. Stuck, A., et al., *A trial of annual in-home comprehensive geriatric assessments for elderly people living in the community*. The New England Journal of Medicine, 1995. **333**(18): p. 1184–1189.

64. Naylor, M.D., et al., *Comprehensive discharge planning and home follow-up of hospitalized elders. A randomized clinical trial*. Journal of the American Medical Association, 1999. **281**: p. 613–620.

65. Krammer, L.M., et al., in *Palliative Care Nursing: Quality Care to the End of Life*, M.L. Matzo and D.W. Sherman, Editors. 2001, Springer Publishing Co: New York.

GENERAL REFERENCES

Adelstein, D.J. (1995). Palliative chemotherapy for non-small cell lung cancer. *Seminars in Oncology, 22(2 Suppl 3)*: 35–39.

Blair, S.N., Kohl, H.W.I., Barlow, E.E., Paffenbarger, R.S., Jr., Gibbons, L.W., & Macera, C.A., (1995). Changes in physical fitness and all-cause mortality: A prospective study of healthy and unhealthy men. *Journal of the American Medical Association, 273(14)*: 1093–1098.

Byock, I. (1997). Why do we make dying so miserable? *The Washington Post*, January 22, 1997.

Gornick, M.E., Warren, J.L., Eggers, P.W., Lubitz, J.D., DeLew, N., Davis, M.H., et al. (1996). Thirty years of medicare: Impact on the covered population. *Health Care Financing Review, 18(2)*: 179–237.

Ferrell, B., Grant, M., Padilla, G., Vemuri, R., Rhine, M. (1990). The experience of pain and perceptions of quality of life: Validation of a conceptual model. *Seminars in Oncology Nursing*, 6(4): 260–270.

Hadley, J. (1982). *More medical care, better health?* Washington, D.C.: The Urban Institute Press.

Hadley, J., Steinberg, E.P., & Feder, J. (1991). Comparison of uninsured and privately insured hospital patients: Condition on admission, resource use, and outcome. *Journal of the American Medical Association, 265(3):* 274–279.

Hing, E. & Bloom, B. (1991). *Long-term care for the functionally dependent elderly. American Journal of Public Health, 81(2):*223–225.

Lurie, N., Ward, N.B., Shapiro, M.F., & Brook, R.H. (1984). Termination from Medi-Cal: Does it affect health? *New England Journal of Medicine, 311*(7): 480–484.

Lurie, N., Ward, N.B., Shapiro, M.R., et al (1986). Termination from Medi-Cal: A follow-up study one year later. *New England Journal of Medicine, 314*(19): 1266–1268.

Manton, K.G., Stallard, E., & Woodbury, M.A. (1994). *Chronic disability trends in elderly United States populations: 1982–1994*. Proceedings of the National Academy of Sciences, 94(6): 2593–2598, 1997. Retrieved at URL http://www.pnas.org/cgi/content/full/94/6/2593.

Pepper Commission (U.S. Bipartisan Commission on Comprehensive Health Care Outcomes). (1990). *A call for action*. Washington, D.C.: U.S. Government Printing Office.

PPRC (Physician Payment Review Commission)(1996). *Annual report to congress.* Washington, D.C.

ProPAC (Prospective Payment Assessment Commission) (1996). *Medicare and the American health care system: Report to the congress.* Washington, D.C.

Vladeck, B.C., & Miller, N.A. (1994). The Medicare home health initiative. *Health Care Financing Review*, 16(1): 7–16.

WHO (World Health Organization). *Cancer pain relief and palliative care.* WHO Technical Report Series 804. Geneva: WHO, 1990.

Chapter XI

Trends for the Future

Patricia Murphy, R.N., M.A.
Betty Rolling Ferrell, Ph.D., F.A.A.N.

I.   Issues Affecting Health Care Delivery in the Next 20 Years

A.   Labor shortages, especially shortages of nursing personnel

1.   By the year 2005 there will be a shortage of 400,000 Registered Nurses in the United States

B.   Increase in chronic disease population

1.   It is anticipated that by 2020 there will be 14 million individuals with Alzheimer's disease as opposed to 4 million in 2001

2.   Other chronic diseases have a similar demographic profile

C.   Increase in population of those over the age of 65

1.   The death rate continues to decline

2.   The median age nationally is 35.3 years, up from 28 years in 1990

3.   Average life expectancy is 74 years for males and 79 years for females

4.   40 million baby boomers will begin to hit the age of 65 in 2009

D.   Healthcare cost containment

1.   In 2000, health care costs were 18% of the gross national product having risen nearly 1% per year over the past decade

2.   One out of eight Medicare dollars is spent on patients in the last three weeks of life

E.   New family structures/Elder caregiver issues

1.   The number of traditional nuclear families has decreased by 3.7% from 1990 to the year 2000

2.   70% of children live in a household where a single parent or both parents are employed outside of the home

3.   The number of individuals living alone is 20.6%, one third of whom are over the age of 65

4.   Nearly 26 million Americans spend an average of 18 hours a week caring for frail relatives or friends suffering from progressive chronic medical conditions

5.   73% of family caregivers are women

F.   Consumer awareness of health and wellness

1.   Consumer advocacy groups have formed in response to managed care cost containment strategies

2.   The media produces more health related public information

3.   60% of WEB users access healthcare information on the Internet

G.   Medicare Trust at risk

1.   Government predictions are that bankruptcy of the Medicare Trust may occur by 2020

H.   Multi-Culturalism

1.   The Nation is becoming more culturally diverse

2.   There was an 11% rise in the Latino population, and 6% rise in Asian in the years from 1990 to 2000

I.   Increasingly sophisticated technology

1.   The utilization of the laser, computerized axial tomography, nuclear magnetic resonance devices, micro-surgery and gene therapy are revolutionizing medicine

2.   Tele-medicine applications such as inter-active video are in use currently with more products being created

J.   Bio-technology/The Genome project

1.   The human genome project is slated to complete its work in 2005 leading to a potential revolution in the modification of disease

K.   Broadened use of Advanced Directives

II. **Goals for Reform of End of Life Care in the 10 Years**

    A. **The development of a cost effective care management model from diagnosis of chronic illness onward that would combine disease modifying therapies, palliative care and hospice**

    B. **Consumer education and public engagement about choice in treatment services and advanced health care directives**

    C. **Education of physicians and other health and human services professionals about clinical, psychological, social, spiritual, cultural, economic and ethical aspects of palliative care and hospice**

    D. **Funding for demonstration projects of new models for end of life care**

    E. **Medicare funding for palliative care and long term care, and continued and enhanced funding of hospice care**

    F. **Applying telemedicine technology to the care process.**

    G. **Bereavement services for survivors**

III. **Actualizing a New Model for Reform of End of Life Care**

    A. **Change will occur as a result of an effective inter-face of public policy, legislation, the development of standards of care, research and adequate reimbursement**

    B. **National Hospice leaders will lead the development of new end of life care models and will advocate for demonstration projects, standards and funding**

    C. **The Federal government will create demonstration projects that will study hospice and palliative care, case management models, long term care models and reimbursement methodologies**

IV. **Legislation as a Component of Reform**

    A. **Major Statements will Guide Reform of End of Life Care**

        1. The SUPPORT Study[1]

            a) Funded by the Robert Wood Johnson Foundation the study focused on decision making and physician practice at the end of life

            b) A major study involving over 9,000 patients in acute care settings with the goal of evaluating end of life care

        2. Institute Of Medicine Report—1997

            a) In 1993, the Institute of Medicare embarked on a survey of end of life care nationwide which culminated in a report that identified steps that can be taken to improve care at the end of life

            b) A consensus document addressing the needs for the nation to improve end of life care

3. National Comprehensive Cancer Network (NCCN) Guidelines for Palliative Care, 2001: leading cancer centers addressing end of life care

4. Institute of Medicine (IOM)/National Cancer Policy Board (NCPB) Report for End of Life Care/Cancer Centers 2001; a consensus document on improving care in cancer centers

5. Institute of Medicine (IOM) Pediatric Report, 2001: Builds on the earlier IOM report to address pediatric needs

6. National Hospice Work Group: Access and Values Project[2]

   a) The NHWG is a group of hospice leaders who convened a series of meetings with influential decision makers to discuss expansion of the hospice model of care into the delivery of palliative care

   b) A consensus project to evaluate the current access and services of hospice and need for reforms

B. **Barriers to Hospice Care will be Lessened**

1. The six-month prognostic requirement will be changed increasing access to hospice for chronically ill individuals nearing life's end

2. The Hospice clinical and leadership model will be fully integrated across the continuum of care into hospitals, nursing homes, daycare and home health care

3. Additional reimbursement will enable hospice to develop palliative care programs for the chronically ill

V. **Reimbursement as a Component of Reform**

A. **The security of the Medicare Trust will be a central goal**

B. **Reimbursement methodology for palliative care and hospice care will reflect innovative care delivery such as case management and telehealth**

C. **Managed care entities will be held to distinct standards for end of life care case management and payment**

D. **Medical groups and third party payer organizations will utilize the most cost effective and ethical end of life care models**

VI. **Standards of Care as a Component of Reform**

A. **The health care industry will apply uniform standards for end of life care across the continuum of care**

B. **A tiered system of centers of excellence in end of life care offering hospice and palliative care will be developed**

C. **Standards and certification for all disciplines involved in end of life care will be developed and promulgated**

D.   Quality end of life care will be measured against clinical performance indicators developed by the hospice industry

E.   Bench marking of individual programs and models that offer end of life care will occur

F.   Education of health care professionals about quality end of life care, including pain management, symptom control, client-family focus, psycho-social spiritual issues, self-determined life closure, case management across the continuum, ethical issues, cultural diversity and communication will occur as part of a program and discipline specific certification initiative nation wide

VII.   **Research as a Component of Reform**

A.   **Research will be identified as a critical component in the development of new models**

B.   **Critical areas of research will be:**

1.   Pain management

2.   Symptom management

3.   Communication

4.   Roles and needs of the primary caregiver

5.   Professional education approaches

6.   Health policy studies

7.   Cost analysis

8.   Bereavement

9.   Effectiveness of varied models of care

10.   Psychosocial and spiritual end of life care

11.   Quality of life closure

VIII.   **Key Partnerships as Component of Reform**

A.   **Provider Organizations**

B.   **Public Interest Groups**

C.   **The Federal and State Governments**

D.   **The Business Community**

E.   **Private Foundations**

F.   **Related Human Service Organizations**

G.   **Health Care Professionals**

H.   **Elder Care Associations and Advocacy Groups**

I.   **The Disabled**

J.   **Multi-Cultural Advocacy Groups**

K.   **Consumer Advocacy**

IX.   **Future Professional Roles in Hospice/Palliative Care**

A.   **Role of Hospice/Palliative Care Certified Nurse**

1.   Skilled assessment, intervention, care coordination, case management and program leadership

2.   Management with the goal of providing care and services to patients with advanced medical illness along the continuum of care in a variety of settings

3.   Supportive care to survivors

4.   Education of consumer and professional community

5.   Support of research and public policy

B.   **Roles for Advanced Practice Nurses (Clinical Nurse Specialist and Nurse Practitioner)**

1.   Primary care model

2.   Utilization of advanced practice skills focused on care and referral to meet comprehensive needs of patients with advanced medical illness

C.   **Roles for nurse researchers prepared at the Doctoral level**

1.   Identification of areas for research in advanced medical illness

2.   Design and implementation of human subject research based on sound clinical practice and ethical principles

3.   Design and implementation of organizational and public policy research to improve systems

D.   **Role of unlicensed personnel**

1.   NBCHPN® certification for Nursing Assistants

2.   Provides physical care that assists activities of daily living and promotes quality of life

3.   Provides emotional support and respite for primary caregivers; assists with nutrition; reports status changes to the RN, NP or CNS

X.   Model Programs

    A.   Models that extend/integrate hospice and palliative care into active treatment

        1.   Project Safe Conduct, a demonstration project, features collaboration between a community-based hospice (Hospice of the Western Reserve) and a NCI cancer center (Ireland Cancer Center of Case Western Reserve University/University Hospitals of Cleveland), which led to pioneering a groundbreaking model of palliative care, funded by the Robert Wood Johnson Foundation

            a)   Project's premise entails vertically integrating the principles of palliative/EOL care into the acute care setting rather than creating a separate team

            b)   Patients are not required to abandon life-prolonging care including experimental therapy protocols in order to receive palliative care

            c)   If treatment fails, a seamless transition occurs from the acute care program to the hospice program. Primary oncologists remain involved through the entire course of the disease

        2.   UC Davis project (Fred Mayers PI)—a model of simultaneous care to integrate palliative care with clinical trials

        3.   Hospice of The Bluegrass—provides palliative care consultation in an inpatient and outpatient setting

    B.   Models integrating palliative care into home care and other settings

        1.   HOPE is a National Cancer Institute funded project (Betty Ferrell PhD, PI) to incorporate palliative care into non-hospice home care settings

        2.   Hospice Palliative Care Center of The North Shore—is a hospital based palliative care unit operated by a certified hospice program

References

1.   SUPPORT, S.P.I., *A controlled trial to improve care for seriously ill hospitalized patients: A study to understand prognoses and preferences for outcomes and risks of treatments (SUPPORT).* Journal of the American Medical Association, 1995. **274**: p. 1591–1598.

2.   Ryndes, T., et al., *Just access and human values in hospice and palliative care: Building an end-of-life care system for the 21st century.* 2001, The Hastings Center and the National Hospice Work Group.

GENERAL REFERENCES

Alexander, C. (1999, Summer). The interface between hospice and palliative care: Observations from a physician. *The Hospice Professional,* 1–4.

American Association of Colleges of Nursing. (1997). Peaceful death: Recommended competencies and curricular guidelines for end-of-life nursing care. *Report from the Robert Wood Johnson End-of-Life Care Roundtable.* Washington, DC.

American Health Decisions. (1997). *The quest to die with dignity.* Appleton, WI: Author.

Byock, I. (1997). *Dying well: The prospect for growth at the end of life.* New York: Riverhead Books.

Chirstakis, N. (1999). *Death foretold.* Chicago: University of Chicago Press.

Ferrell, B., Virani, R., Grant, M., Coyne, P., Uman, G. (2000). Beyond the Supreme Court decision: Nursing perspectives on end-of-life care. *Oncology Nursing Forum,* 27(3): 445–455.

Ferrell, B., Virani, R., Grant, M. (1999). Analysis of end-of-life content in nursing textbooks. *Oncology Nursing Forum,* 26(5): 869–876.

Ferrell, B.R., Grant, M., & Virani, R. (1999). Strengthening nursing education to improve end of life care. *Nursing Outlook,* **47**: 252–256.

Field, M.J., Cassell, C.K., (Eds.) (1997). Approaching death: Improving care at the end of life. *Report of the Institute of Medicine Task Force.* Washington, D.C.: National Academy Press.

Lynn, J. (1996). Caring at the end of our lives. *New England Journal of Medicine,* 335: 210–202.

National Hospice and Palliative Care Organization (1999), *Medicare benefit reform task force report.* Alexandria, VA: Author.

McCaffery, M., Ferrell, B. (1997). Nurses' knowledge of pain assessment and management: How much progress have we made? *Journal of Pain and Symptom Management* 10: 356–367.

Miller, S., et al. (2000, March). *Synthesis and analysis of Medicare's hospice benefit: Executive summary and recommendations.* Washington, DC: United States Department of Health and Human Services.

Rabow, M.W., Hardie, G.E., Fair, J.M., McPhee, S.J. (2000). End-of-life care: Content in 50 textbooks from multiple specialties. *Journal of the American Medical Association,* 283(6): 771–778.

Schulz, R. & Beach, S.R. (1999). Caregiving as a risk factor for mortality: The caregiver health effects study. *Journal of the American Medical Association* 282: 2215–2219.

Webb, M. (1997). *The good death: The new American search to reshape the end of life.* New York. Bantam Books.

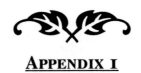

APPENDIX I

WEBSITE/INTERNET RESOURCES*

Agency for Healthcare Research and Quality	http://www.ahcpr.gov/
Aging with Dignity	http://www.agingwithdignity.org
American Academy of Hospice and Palliative Medicine	http://www.aahpm.org
American Academy of Pain Medicine	http://www.painmed.org
American Association for Therapeutic Humor	http://www.aath.org
ABCD Americans for Better Care of the Dying	http://www.abcd-caring.com
American Board of Internal Medicine— Care for the Dying, Physician Narratives	http://www.abim.org/pubs/narr001.htm
American Cancer Society	http://www.cancer.org
American Chronic Pain Association	http://www.theacpa.org/
American Council for Headache Education	http://www.achenet.org
The American Geriatrics Society	http://www.americangeriatrics.org
American Holistic Nurses Association	http://www.ahna.org
American Massage Therapy Association	http://www.amtamassage.org
American Medical Association	http://www.ama-assn.org.80/about.htm
American Medical Association Education of Physicians on End of Life Care (EPEC)	http://www.ama-assn.org/ama/pub/category/2719.html
American Music Therapy Association	http://www.namt.com
American Pain Foundation	http://www.painfoundation.org
American Pain Society	http://www.ampainsoc.org
American Society of Anesthesiologists	http://www.asahq.org
American Society for Bioethics and Humanities	http://www.asbh.org
American Society of Clinical Oncology (ASCO)	http://www.asco.org
American Society of Law, Medicine and Ethics	http://www.aslme.org
American Society of Pain Management Nurses	http://www.aspmn.org

---

* From TEXTBOOK OF PALLIATIVE NURSING, edited by Betty Ferrell and Nessa Coyle, copyright–2000 by Oxford University Press, Inc. Used by permission of Oxford University Press, Inc.

Editor's Note: Any URLs found to be non-functional or inaccurate at the time of publication have been either corrected or deleted.

Approaching Death: Improving Care at the End of Life	http://www.nap.edu/readingroom/books/approaching/
Arthritis Foundation	http://www.arthritis.org
Association of Cancer Online Resources, Inc.	http://www.acor.org
Association of American Sickle Cell Disease	http://www.sicklecelldisease.org
Association of Death Education and Counseling (ADEC)	http://www.adec.org
Association of Nurses in AIDS Care	http://www.anacnet.org
Association of Oncology Social Work (AOSW)	http://www.aosw.org
Association of Pediatric Oncology Nurses (APON)	http://www.apon.org
Before I Die: Medical Care and Personal Choices	http://www.wnet.org/archive/bid
Bereavement and Hospice Support Netline	http://www.ubalt.edu/www/bereavement
Cancer Care, Inc.	http://www.cancercare.org
Cancer Links	http://www.personal.u-net.com/~njh/cancer.html
Cancer Net	http://www.cancernet.nci.nih.gov/
Candlelighters Childhood Cancer Foundation	http://www.candlelighters.org
Caregiver Network	http://www.caregiver.on.ca/index.html
Caregiver Survival Resources	http://www.caregiver911.com/
Catholic Health Association of the United States	http://www.chausa.org
Center for Medical Ethics and Mediation	http://www.cmem.org/
Center to Improve Care of the Dying	http://www.gwu.edu/~cicd
Children's Hospice International	http://www.chionline.org
Choice in Dying	http://www.choices.org
City of Hope Pain/Palliative Care Resource Center	http://prc.coh.org
The Compassionate Friends	http://www.compassionatefriends.org/
Compassion in Dying	http://www.compassionindying.org
C. Richard Chapman Pain Information Page	http://faculty.washington.edu/crc/
Cultural Guides to Dying, Death & the Afterlife	http://www.indranet.com/bardo/cultural.html
Department of Health and Human Services, Healthfinder	http://www.healthfinder.gov
Dying Well	http://www.dyingwell.org or http://www.dyingwell.com
The Edmonton Palliative Care Program	http://www.palliative.org
Education for Physicians on End of Life Care Project (EPEC)	http://www.epec.net
The End of Life: Exploring Death in America	http://www.npr.org/programs/death/
End of Life Physician Education Resource Center (EPERC)	http://www.eperc.mcw.edu
FACCT—The Foundation for Accountability	http://www.facct.org
Family Caregiver Alliance	http://www.caregiver.org
Fibromyalgia Network	http://www.fmnetnews.com

Growth House	http://www.growthhouse.org
Hospice Association of America	http://www.hospice-america.org
Hospice and Palliative Nurses Association	http://www.hpna.org
Hospice Foundation of America	http://www.hospicefoundation.org
Hospice Hands	http://www.hospice-cares.com
Institute for Healthcare Improvement	http://www.ihi.org
International Association for the Study of Pain	http://www.iasp-pain.org/
Last Acts	http://www.lastacts.org
Leukemia Society of America	http://www.leukemia.org
Make a Wish Foundation	http://www.wish.org
Management of Cancer Pain	http://www.ahcpr.gov/consumer/
Medical College of Wisconsin Bioethics	http://www.mcw.edu/bioethics/
Medical College of Wisconsin Palliative Care Program	http://www.mcw.edu/pallmed/
Memorial Sloan-Kettering Cancer Center	http://www.mskcc.org
The Nathan Cummings Foundation	http://www.ncf.org/index.html
National Association for Home Care (NAHC)	http://www.nahc.org/
The National Center for Health Statistics	http://www.cdc.gov/nchs/about.htm
National Conference of State Legislatures	http://www.ncsl.org/programs/pubs/endoflife.htm
National Family Caregivers Association	http://www.nfcacares.org/
National Hospice and Palliative Care Organization	http://www.nhpco.org
The National Institute of Aging	http://www.nih.gov/nia/
National Prison Hospice Association— Development of Hospice Care in Correctional Facilities	http://www.npha.org
Neuropathy Association	http://www.neuropathy.org
New York State Partnership for Long-Term Care	http://www.nyspltc.org/about/index.html#3
Not Dead Yet	http://www.notdeadyet.org/
On Our Own Terms	http://www.thirteen.org/onourownterms
Oncolink	http://www.oncolink.com
Oncolinks Pain Page	http://oncolink.upenn.edu/specialty/pain
Open Society Institute Project on Death in America	http://www.soros.org/death.html
Oregon Health Sciences University Center for Ethics in Health Care	http://www.ohsu.edu/ethics/
Oncology Nursing Society	http://www.ons.org
Pain Link	http://www.edc.org/PainLink
Pain Net	http://www.painnet.com
The Palliative Medicine Program	http://www.mcw.edu/pallmed
Partners Against Pain	http://www.partnersagainstpain.com
The Patient Education Institute	http://www.patient-education.com

Pediatric Pain	http://is.dal.ca/~pedpain/prohp.html
Pediatric Pain Education for Patients & Families	http://pedspain.nursing.uiowa.edu/resources/kids.htm
Project on Death in America	http://www.soros.org/death/
Reflex Sympathetic Dystrophy Association of California	http://www.rsdsa-ca.org/
Resource Center of the American Alliance Of Cancer Pain Initiatives	http://www.aacpi.org/resource.html
The Robert Wood Johnson Foundation	http://www.rwjf.org
Roxane Pain Institute	http://pain.roxane.com
Southern California Cancer Pain Initiative (SCCPI)	http://sccpi.coh.org
Supportive Care of the Dying	http://www.careofdying.org
TMJ Association, Ltd.	http://www.tmj.org
Talarian Map-Cancer Pain	http://www.stat.washington.edu/TALARIA/talariahome.html
Telemedicine Information Exchange	http://tie.telemed.org
United Hospital Fund of New York	http://www.uhfnyc.org
University of Wisconsin Pain & Policy Studies Group	http://www.medsch.wisc.edu/painpolicy/
VistaCare	http://www.vista-care.com
Wellness Web Cancer Center	http://www.wellnessweb.com/CANCER/cancer.htm
When Death is Sought Assisted Suicide and Euthanasia in the Medical Context	http://www.health.state.ny.us/nysdoh/provider/death.htm
Wisconsin Cancer Pain Initiative	http://www.wisc.edu/wcpi
Worldwide Congress on Pain	http://www.careofdying.org

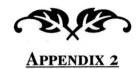

COMMONLY USED MEDICATIONS
Trade And Generic Names*

ANTIFUNGAL

Mycelex®, Lotrimin® . . . . clotrimazole
Nizoral® . . . . ketoconazole
Flagyl® . . . . metronidazole
Monistat® . . . . miconazole nitrate
Diflucan® . . . . fluconazole
Sporonox® . . . . itraconazole

ANTIGOUT

Zyloprim®, Lopurin® . . . . allopurinol
Benemid® . . . . probenecid
Colchicine MR®, Colgout® . . . . colchicine

ANXIOLYTIC

Ativan® . . . . lorazepam
Tranxene® . . . . clorazepate
BuSpar® . . . . buspirone
Sinequan®, Adapin® . . . . doxepin
Librium® . . . . chlordiazepoxide HCL
Valium® . . . . diazepam

ANTIHISTAMINES

Atarax® . . . . hydroxyzine HCL
Benadryl® . . . . diphenhydramine HCL
Chlor-trimeton® . . . . chlorpheniramine
Allegra® . . . . fexofenadine
Claritin® . . . . loratadine
Tavist® . . . . clemastine fumarate

* Source: *Drug Facts and Comparisons*®. (November, 2001). St. Louis: A Wolters Kluwer Company.

ANTIANGINAL

Isordil® . . . . isosorbide
Procardia® . . . . nifedipine
Calan®, Isoptin® . . . . verapamil
Persantine® . . . . dipyridamole
Nitro-Bid® . . . . nitroglycerine

ANTIPRURITICS

Caladryl® . . . . calamine & diphenhydramine

ANTINAUSEANTS/ANTIEMETICS/PRO-MOTILITY

Antivert® . . . . meclizine HCL
Compazine® . . . . prochlorperazine
Dramamine® . . . . dimenhydrinate
Phenergan® . . . . promethazine HCL
Thorazine® . . . . chlorpromazine HCL
Tigan® . . . . trimethobenzamide HCL
Torecan® . . . . triethylperazine
Reglan® . . . . metoclopramide HCL

ANALGESICS

Actiq® . . . . fentanyl citrate
Darvocet N® . . . . propoxyphene napsylate w/acetaminophen
Darvon® . . . . propoxyphene HCL
Demerol® . . . . meperidine HCL
Dilaudid® . . . . hydromorphone HCL
Dolophine® . . . . methadone HCL
Duragesic® . . . . fentanyl transdermal system
Empirin w/Codeine® . . . . ASA w/codeine
Fiorinal® . . . . butalbital w/ASA & caffeine
MS Contin® . . . . morphine sulfate
Oramorph® SR. . . . . morphine sulfate
Oxycontin® . . . . oxycodone
Percocet®, Roxicet® . . . . oxycodone w/acetaminophen
Percodan® . . . . oxycodone w/ASA
Roxanol® . . . . morphine sulfate
Talwin® . . . . pentazocine HCL
Tylenol w/Codeine® . . . . APAP w/codeine

ANTACIDS/ANTIFLATULANTS/DIGESTANTS

Basaljel®. . . . . aluminum carbonate gel
Gelusil® . . . . aluminum hydroxide
Maalox® . . . . magnesium hydroxide & aluminum hydroxide
Mylanta® . . . . magnesium hydroxide & aluminum hydroxide & simethicone
Mylicon® . . . . simethicone
Pancrease® . . . . pancrelipase
Viokase® . . . . pancreatin

BETA-ADRENERGIC BLOCKERS

Corgard® . . . . nadolol
Inderal® . . . . .propranolol
Tenormin® . . . . .atenolol
Trandate® . . . . .labetalol HCL
Lopressor® . . . . .metoprolol

ALZHEIMER'S DRUGS

Cognex® . . . . .tacrine HCL
Aricept® . . . . .donepezil

ANTIDEPRESSANTS

Adapin®, Sinequan® . . . . .doxepin HCL
Elavil®, Endep® . . . . .amitriptyline HCL
Norpramin® . . . . .desipramine HCL
Pamelor® . . . . .nortriptyline HCL
Surmontil® . . . . .trimipramine
Tofranil® . . . . .imipramine HCL
Tofranil PM® . . . . .imipramine pamoate
Vivactil®. . . . . .protryptyline HCL
Mirzataprine® . . . . .remuron
Desyrel® . . . . .trazodone HCL
Wellbutrin® . . . . .bupropion HCL
Effexor® . . . . .venlafaxine HCL
Serzone® . . . . .nefazodone HCL
Prozac® . . . . .fluoxetine HCL
Luvox® . . . . fluvoxamine
Paxil® . . . . paroxetine HCL
Zoloft® . . . . sertraline HCL

ANXIOLYTIC & ANTIDEPRESSANT COMBINATONS

Etrafon®, Triavil® . . . . perphenazine & amitriptyline
Limbitrol® . . . . chlordiazepoxide & amitriptyline

MAJOR TRANQUILIZERS

Butyrophenones:
Haldol®. . . . . haloperidol
Phenothiazines:
Mellaril® . . . . thioridazine HCL
Prolixin® . . . . fluphenazine
Thorazine® . . . . chlorpromazine HCL
Trilafon® . . . . perphenazine

MUSCLE RELAXANTS

Flexeril® . . . . cyclobenzaprine HCL
Quinamm® . . . . quinine sulfate
Valium®, Valrelease® . . . . diazepam
Lioresal®. . . . . baclofen
Robaxin® . . . . methocarbamol
Norflex® . . . . orphenadrine

SEDATIVE/HYPNOTICS

Nembutal® . . . . pentobarbital
Seconal® . . . . secobarbital
Dalmane® . . . . flurazepam HCL
Halcion® . . . . triazolam
Placidyl® . . . . ethchlorvynol
Restoril® . . . . temazepam
Ambien® . . . . zolpidem

ANTIDIARRHEAL

Donnagel® . . . . kaolin & pectin (OTC)
Imodium® . . . . loperamide (OTC)
Kaopectate® . . . . kaolin & pectin (OTC)
Lomotil® . . . . diphenoxylate & atropine
Paregoric® . . . . camphorated opium tincture (contains morphine)
Pepto-Bismol® . . . . bismuth subsalicylate (OTC)

ANTIPSYCHOTICS

Moban® . . . . molindone HCL
Loxitane® . . . . loxapine HCL
Clozaril® . . . . clozapine
Risperdal® . . . . risperidone
Zyprexa® . . . . olanzapine
Stelazine® . . . . trifluoperazine
Navane® . . . . thiothixene
Seroquel® . . . . quetiapine

ANTICONVULSANTS

Tegretol® . . . . carbamazepine
Dilantin® . . . . phenytoin
Depakote® . . . . valproic acid
Klonopin® . . . . clonazepam
Neurontin® . . . . gabapentin

MISCELLANEOUS

Aredia® . . . . pamidronate
Sandostatin® . . . . octreotide
Zovirax® . . . . acyclovir
Colace®, Surfak®, Regutol® . . . . docusate sodium
Valtrex® . . . . valacyclovir

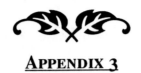

STANDARDS OF HOSPICE CARE FOR CHILDREN*

Access to Care

> * **Principle:** Children with life-threatening illnesses and their families have special needs. Hospice services for children and their families offer developmentally appropriate palliative and supportive care to any child with a life-threatening condition in any appropriate setting. Children are admitted to hospice services without regard for diagnosis, gender, race, creed, handicap, age, or ability to pay.

> * **Standards:**

>> **A.C.1.** Hospice care services are accessible to children and their families in a setting that is desired and/or appropriate for their needs.

>> **A.C.2.** The hospice team is available to provide continuity of care to children and their families in the home and/or in an institutional setting

>> **A.C.3.** The hospice program has eligibility admission criteria for the children and families they serve. Care plans are developed which take into consideration the child's prognosis and the child and families needs and desires for hospice services. Admission to the hospice care services does not preclude the child and the family from treatment choices or hopeful, supportive therapies.

>> **A.C.4.** The hospice program provides information to the community and referral sources about the services that are offered, who qualifies, and how services may be obtained and reimbursed.

Child and Family as a Unit of Care

> * **Principle:** Hospice programs provide family-centered care to enhance the quality of life for the children and family as defined by each child-and family unit. It includes the child and family in the decision-making process about services and treatment choices to the fullest degree that is possible and desired.

> * **Standards:**

>> C.F.U.1. The unit of care is child and family. Hospice provides family-centered care. The family is defined as the relatives and/or other significant persons who provide physical, psychological, social, and/or spiritual support for the child.

---

* Quoted with permission: Children's Hospice International. (1993) *Standards of hospice care for children.* Retrieved October 31, 2001, from http://www.chionline.org/standards.html

C.F.U.2. The hospice program recognizes the unique, personal values and beliefs of all children and families. The hospice respects and maintains, as possible, the wishes and dignity of every child and his or her family.

C.F.U.3. The hospice program encourages that children and their families participate in decisions regarding care, including discontinuation of hospice care at any time, and maintains documentation related to consent, advance directives, treatments, and alternative choices of care.

C.F.U.4. The hospice program provides care that considers each child's growth, development and stage of family life cycle. Children's interests and needs are solicited and considered, but are not limited to those related to their illness and disability.

C.F.U.5. The hospice seeks to assist each child and family to enjoy life as they are able, and to continue in their customary life-style, functioning and roles as much as possible, especially helping the child to live a normal life as is possible.

Policies and Procedures

* **Principle:** The hospice program offers services that are accountable to and appropriate for the children and families it serves.

* **Standards:**

  P.P.1. The hospice program establishes and maintains accurate and adequate policies and procedures to assure that the hospice is accountable to children, their families, and the communities they serve.

  P.P.2. The hospice agency is in compliance with all local, state and federal laws and regulations that govern the appropriate delivery of hospice care services.

  P.P.3. The hospice program provides a clear and accessible grievance procedure to families outlining how to voice complaints or concerns about services and care without jeopardizing services.

Interdisciplinary Team Services

* **Principle:** Seriously ill children with life-threatening conditions and/or facing terminal stages of an illness and their families have a variety of needs that require a collaborative and cooperative effort from practitioners of many disciplines, working together as an interdisciplinary team of qualified professionals and volunteers.

* **Standards:**

  I.T.1. The hospice program provides care to the child and family by utilizing a core interdisciplinary team which may include: the child, the family and/or significant others, physicians, nurses, social workers, clergy, and volunteers.

  I.T.2. Representatives of other appropriate disciplines are involved in the team as needed, i.e., physical therapy, occupational therapy, speech therapy, nutritional consultation, art therapy, music therapy. The team might also include psychologists, child life specialists, teachers, recreation therapists, play therapists, home health aides, nursing assistants, and other specialists or services as needed.

  I.T.3. The hospice core team meets on a regular basis and an integrated plan of care is developed, implemented and maintained for every child and family.

I.T.4. The hospice staff professionals are qualified in their particular discipline by training, experience, certification and/or licensure. Complete orientation, training and continuing education are provided to each hospice staff member.

I.T.5. The hospice has an active volunteer program. All volunteers are carefully and appropriately selected, trained, supervised and evaluated, at least annually, by hospice professionals.

I.T.6. All hospice personnel receive educational, psychological and emotional support appropriate to their situations needs and desires.

I.T.7. The hospice core interdisciplinary team meets at least every two weeks or sooner if needed to review and update all plans of care.

Continuity of Care

* **Principle:** Hospice is an integrated system of home and inpatient care. Hospice provides a consistent continuum of care in all settings from when admitted to the end of bereavement services.

* **Standards:**

C.C.1. Hospice services are available to children and their families on a consistent basis: seven days a week and 24 hours a day institutions or at home.

C.C.2. Appropriate hospice team members are available to children and their families on an on-call basis when the office is closed.

C.C.3. The hospice program has a communication system that assures confidentiality and privacy, and can be used to update team members about each child and family's status so that needs can be addressed as soon as possible.

C.C.4. All children and families receive a timely and comprehensive assessment of their physical, psychosocial, emotional, spiritual, and financial needs.

C.C.5. The hospice team, with the family, develops and integrated, written, interdisciplinary plan of care for each child and family. The plan addresses the unique and individual needs of the child and family including: assessment, identified present and potential problems, interventions and the type and level of services to be provided.

C.C.6. The hospice team addresses and documents the concerns, needs, and desires of the child and family in developing and implementing the plan of care. This document is updated as indicated by the changing status of the child or family.

C.C.7. The hospice agency maintains appropriate documents and clinical records. The clinical record includes properly executed consents for medical/hospice treatment. Confidentiality of hospice records is maintained.

Pain and Symptom Management

* **Principle:** Children should be as symptom-free as possible, and pain and/or other symptoms of their illness should be managed to achieve the greatest possible comfort.

* **Standards:**

P.S.M.1. The hospice team assists the children in achieving comfort through the most effective treatments available.

P.S.M.2 Palliative therapies are discussed with children and their families and provided to children to ensure the most effective and adequate pain symptom management.

P.S.M.3. Alternative methods of pain and symptom management are discussed and incorporated into care of the child as appropriate.

Bereavement Program

* **Principle:** Families of children who die may continue to need appropriate professional and supportive services for a period following death

* **Standards:**

B.P.1. The hospice program has a structured active bereavement program. Bereavement services are provided to the surviving family member's and/or significant others. Special attention may need to be given to siblings who may not be able to articulate their needs for support.

B.P.2. The level and type of services provided are determined by the family member(s) and appropriate hospice team members.

B.P.3. Bereavement services are available and provided for at least thirteen months following the death of the child, extending throughout the second year if possible.

Utilization Review/Quality Improvement

* **Principle:** The hospice program should monitor and ensure the appropriate allocation and utilization of resources and effectiveness of services.

* **Standards:**

U.R.1. The hospice program has a written continuous quality improvement and utilization review program. The program includes criteria to assess the overall functioning components of the hospice program and the effectiveness of its services.

U.R.2. The continuous quality improvement and utilization review program is an ongoing process and implemented on a regular basis with results of the evaluation that are reported to appropriate individuals and/or committees for action.

U.R.3. The hospice program provides a written evaluation tool for all recipients of services to document their satisfaction or dissatisfaction with the services received. A written plan outlining how evaluation information will be used to improve services is available to all consumers.

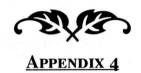

STANDARDS OF HOSPICE NURSING PRACTICE AND PROFESSIONAL PERFORMANCE*

Standards of Hospice Nursing Practice:

Standard I.   **Assessment:**
THE HOSPICE NURSE COLLECTS PATIENT AND FAMILY DATA

Standard II.   **Diagnosis:**
THE HOSPICE NURSE ANALYZES THE ASSESSMENT DATA IN DETERMINING DIAGNOSIS

Standard III.   **Outcome Identification:**
THE HOSPICE NURSE IDENTIFIES EXPECTED OUTCOMES NDIVIDUALIZED TO THE PATIENT AND FAMILY

Standard IV.   **Planning:**
THE HOSPICE NURSE DEVELOPS A NURSING PLAN OF CARE THE PRESCRIBES INTERVENTIONS TO ATTAIN EXPECTED OUTCOMES

Standard V.   **Implementation:**
THE HOSPICE NURSE IMPLEMENTS THE INTERVENTIONS IDENTIFIED IN THE PLAN OF CARE

Standard VI.   **Evaluation:**
THE HOSPICE NURSE EVALUATES THE PATIENT'S AND FAMILY'S PROGRESS TOWARD ATTAINMENT OF OUTCOMES

---

* Used with permission. Hospice Nurses Association Standards and Accreditation Committee. (1995). *Standards of hospice nursing practice and professional performance.* Pittsburgh: PA. Hospice Nurses Association.

Standards of Professional Performance:

Standard I.   **Quality of Care:**
THE HOSPICE NURSE SYSTEMATICALLY EVALUATES THE QUALITY AND EFFECTIVENESS OF NURSING PRACTICE

Standard II.   **Performance Appraisal:**
THE HOSPICE NURSE EVALUATES HIS/HER OWN NURSING PRACTICE IN RELATION TO PROFESSIONAL PRACTICE STANDARDS AND RELEVANT STANDARDS AND REGULATIONS

Standard III.   **Education:**
THE HOSPICE NURSE ACQUIRES AND MAINTAINS CURRENT KNOWLEDGE IN HOSPICE NURSING PRACTICE

Standard IV.   **Collegiality:**
THE HOSPICE NURSE CONTRIBUTES TO THE PROFESSIONAL DEVELOPMENT OF PEERS, COLLEAGUES AND OTHERS

Standard V.   **Ethics:**
THE HOSPICE NURSE'S DECISIONS AND ACTIONS ON BEHALF OF PATIENT AND FAMILY ARE DETERMINED IN AN ETHICAL MANNER

Standard VI.   **Collaboration:**
THE HOSPICE NURSE COLLABORATES WITH THE PATIENT AND FAMILY, OTHER MEMBERS OF THE INTERDISCIPLINARY TEAM, AND OTHER HEALTH CARE PROVIDERS IN PROVIDING PATIENT AND FAMILY CARE

Standard VII.   **Research:**
THE HOSPICE NURSE USES RESEARCH FINDINGS IN PRACTICE.

Standard VIII.   **Resource Utilization:**
THE HOSPICE NURSE CONSIDERS FACTORS RELATED TO SAFETY, EFFECTIVENESS, AND COST IN PLANNING AND DELIVERING PATIENT AND FAMILY CARE